BREATHING SHOULD NEVER BE HARD WORK

One Man's Journey with Idiopathic Pulmonary Fibrosis

Robert Davidson

Cover cartoon illustration drawn by:
Patricia Wheeler
Markham, Ontario

Produced by:

FriesenPress
Suite 300 – 852 Fort Street
Victoria, BC, Canada V8W 1H8

www.friesenpress.com

Distributed to the trade by The Ingram Book Company

Breathing Should Never Be Hard Work

I was inspired to share my journey with Idiopathic Pulmonary Fibrosis because I wanted to be a source of encouragement and help for those suffering from this awful disease. It was surprisingly fun and also quite moving to relive that time. I will never forget the support that I received from family, friends, and the medical professionals, and I will always keep the courage of those waiting for new lungs close to my heart.

Pulmonary Fibrosis continues to kill people all over the world, but there is hope. Thousands of researchers worldwide are now aggressively seeking out causes and treatments. I really believe those treatments will come in my lifetime.

There are some people I would like to thank for their help in writing my story:

My wife, Heather, who supported me through my best and worst days. She kept me going while suffering herself as she watched me dying, and she still supports me by doing all the hard work on the Foundation.

My sons, Mark and Matthew, who also supported me all the way. They also work hard for the Foundation.

Robert Alloway, friend and author, for helping me understand how to start the book.

Eileen Rees, my friend who did such a fine job of editing the work and making the book readable. Without her work, this would just be a list of uninspiring facts with the occasional bit of humour. Eileen made it flow.

Dr Dancey, my respirologist and the rest of the medical staff at Toronto General Hospital; these people, through their great skills and care, made it possible for me to be here to write the story.

MOST OF ALL
MY HERO

My Donor: This caring man or woman selflessly made the choice to sign an organ donor card in order to donate their life-giving organs in the tragic event of their own demise. He or she saved not just my life, but possibly seven others. Without this gift I would not have survived to write this book or to provide support to others.

I hope the donor's family truly understands the magnitude of their gift. Words cannot express our appreciation for how they honoured the donor's final wishes. This kind and generous person was a true hero in every sense of the word.

I would like to encourage all of my readers to follow my donor's example by signing up (if you are in Ontario) at Beadonor.ca. If you're outside of Ontario, you can learn how to be a donor by searching "organ donation (your province/state)" on the Internet.

Breathing Should Never Be Hard Work

My Journey with Idiopathic Pulmonary Fibrosis

Table of Contents

In the Beginning **The Short Version**

"Well, my friend, you have Pulmonary Fibrosis."

Those seven words forever changed my life in ways I could never have even imagined at the time. When my respirologist gave me the diagnosis in October 2007, nothing in my previous 60 years of experience had remotely prepared me for what lay ahead. The journey was, in a word, surreal.

I had never heard of Pulmonary Fibrosis and had no idea what the diagnosis meant, though Dr. Dancey certainly got my attention with the following warning: "If you look it up on the Internet, you'll scare yourself to death."

My wife's reaction to the news was equally comforting:

"Oh my God, that's what killed Janice," said Heather. Her friend's condition had deteriorated rapidly, and she had died very quickly a couple of years earlier while waiting for a lung biopsy.

Well, I *did* look it up on the Internet, and while I didn't scare myself to death, I found that there was no known cause for Idiopathic Pulmonary Fibrosis (IPF), there was only limited treatment and no cure. The prognosis was grim: death within an average of three to five years of diagnosis.

However, I also noticed that a few people lived for 18 years. I'm an accountant, I'm good with numbers; I went with the 18-year option.

> *"Life is what happens to you while you're busy making other plans."*
> - John Lennon

As Robbie Burns said, the best laid schemes of mice and men often go awry, and sure enough, my plans only lasted a couple of years. Pulmonary Fibrosis is an unpredictable disease with many factors beyond our immediate control. Simple things like the common cold can accelerate the symptoms, and once scarring of the lung occurs it is irreversible. A little more breath will be stolen away, and will be gone forever.

In January 2009, less than 15 months after my diagnosis, I caught a minor cold , and the Pulmonary Fibrosis really showed itself. My capacity for exercise was down noticeably, which was a real blow considering I had just come through a year when I barely noticed any symptoms at all. I had continued to referee high-level soccer, even after I'd had a minor heart attack at the USA Soccer Cup. I realised that I needed to avoid people with colds and flu, but that's a real challenge unless you live like Howard Hughes. Clearly, I had to be more vigilant, or else I'd suffer the consequences.

The sharp downturn in my health did get me thinking seriously about my Bucket List, and to press on with establishing the Canadian Pulmonary Fibrosis Foundation (CPFF). I had felt for some time that we needed an information and support network for Canadian Pulmonary Fibrosis patients. It was no mean feat, given the bureaucracy involved, but by October the CPFF was a reality.

I got a head start on the travel section of the Bucket List during that spring and summer. In May, my friend Clyde and I went to Yunnan province in China; in July, I made a return trip to Minnesota for the 25thAnniversary of the USA Soccer Cup, and in August, Heather and I celebrated her 60th birthday in Scotland. One might say that this was a good beginning, but I did notice that I had lost a bit more lung power; I optimistically speculated that it was possibly due to the high altitudes in China. We were up at 12,800 feet near the Tibetan border, in the foothills of the Himalayas. Then again, perhaps it really was just IPF asserting itself. We'll never know for sure, but I do know I really enjoyed those trips, and we created memories to last a lifetime.

In November 2009, just two years after the diagnosis, another cold made me oxygen-dependent as the fibrosis got worse. Now I stumbled around at home, dragging along my 50-foot lifeline. Trips to the pub were only possible courtesy of a small bottle of oxygen, which was good for about 90 minutes, just enough time for a couple of beers with my friends before I needed to get back to Home Sweet Home.

Stairs were a real problem. I had to place chairs halfway up the stairs at my office and at home so that I could rest on the way up. And yes, I sometimes napped during working hours. I had a line of chairs placed six feet apart, between the living room couch and the washroom, like a trail of breadcrumbs. Believe me, six feet can seem endless. I was shocked at how quickly this disease could move.

By December I needed a wheelchair to visit the mall for Christmas shopping. A visit to the public washroom left me so breathless that I could barely stand up. It was on this trip to the mall that I had my first panic attack, I felt like I was about to pass out from a lack of oxygen. It was probably the ignominy of the location that averted that drama.

Just standing up was hard enough now, never mind attempting to do anything else. I brushed my teeth and shaved sitting down while I watched the morning news on TV. I felt instinctively that no matter what it took, it was absolutely vital to preserve as much normalcy as possible in my everyday life so that I wouldn't just give up.

Over Christmas, I got another cold and this was The Big One. Mister IPF took complete control. I had lost over 70 pounds, and my skin was grey. I bore more than a passing resemblance to "The Ghost of Christmas Past" from Dickens's *Christmas Carol*. I felt sorry for friends and family visiting over that period as I'm sure they believed my days were numbered.

Unable to breathe, I paid a Christmas Eve visit to the local hospital. This development alarmed Dr. Dancey enough for him to push Toronto General Lung Transplant Unit to expedite my place on the waiting list for new lungs. He called the evening of December 28th to say that while they were still waiting for the results of one heart test, I was to stop taking my blood thinner medication, a strong indication that I would get listed. After all, surgeons aren't at all keen on seeing too much blood running freely while they cut into you.

On January 19, 2010, we met with Dr. Pierre, a thoracic surgeon, who asked a lot of pointed questions and explained all the details and inherent risks of a transplant. Ten per cent of patients don't survive the operation. That means 90 per cent do! Good odds, I'd say. I had to sign numerous consent and release forms, figuring that it was best do it while I was waiting, because it's low on the priority list after getting the call for a transplant.

A mere 10 days later, at 12:23 AM on January 30th, we got "the call." We had been offered lungs. We arrived at the hospital at 1:40 AM, 77 minutes after getting the call.

After waiting all night while they made sure the lungs were safe to transplant, I finally underwent an eight-hour operation while my family waited outside for news. It must have been tough for them, and it was worse for my youngest son living in Germany; Matthew kept phoning throughout the night for updates. It was fine for me: I slept through the whole thing.

After I woke up in the ICU, and they removed the tube helping me breathe, I could suddenly breathe on my own. What an indescribable feeling after the months when I felt like I was literally suffocating every single day. The breathing was just happening *all by itself!*

Twelve days later I was out of hospital, 22 days from listing to discharge! How about that? I felt a bit guilty about those patients who had been on the list for much longer; some of them waiting for up to three years. I needn't have worried; it turned out that they were just happy for me, and it also gave them fresh hope.

Breathing was so beautiful now, and I threw myself into carrying out the work of the Foundation with renewed energy and purpose. Other people deserve what I have, and hopefully one day they won't need a lung transplant to get there. We *must* find a cure.

Chapter 2 **The Diagnosis**

My diagnosis took some time because Pulmonary Fibrosis has symptoms and an underlying pattern of scarring that can mimic that of other lung disorders. It is difficult to determine, and many people die before even getting on to the transplant list.

I am a soccer referee and had achieved a fairly high standing in Ontario, refereeing senior competitive men's and women's games and the occasional semi-pro game. I had achieved Level 1 status but was now on my way down. Age can do that to you.

At this level, there is a requirement to pass annual fitness tests to retain the grade and continue refereeing the most challenging games. We always completed the test before the season start, and May 27 was the designated day in 2007. It was an auspicious Sunday as it was the day of our 35th wedding anniversary. I had turned 60 just three days before.

The test is quite challenging, requiring two 60-metre sprints in less than eight seconds each, followed by two 200-metre sprints to be completed in less than 35 seconds each, and a 12-minute non-stop run for a minimum of 2,700 metres. I was okay on the sprints but found the 12-minute run really difficult. I hate long-distance running. We never run for 12 minutes straight in a game anyway. I did pass the test and retained my grade for another year but the next morning I had real trouble breathing and coughed up a little blood which was fairly alarming. A quick visit to my family doctor seemed indicated.

She's an excellent doctor, and always seems to know when I should see a specialist. After sending me for x-rays of my lungs she quickly made me an appointment to see a respirologist. Dr. Dancey couldn't see me until September, so he asked me to get an updated x-ray done beforehand for comparison purposes.

After my first appointment, he sent me off for a CT scan and pulmonary function tests, where I was asked to blow into a machine in a variety of different ways. I also did a six- minute walk test where they see how far you can go in the allotted time while they monitor oxygen saturation. I found out some time later that while it is a very simple test, it is also the best test of pulmonary function deterioration.

I carried on refereeing during this period. Hey, I wasn't going to let all that hard work passing the fitness test go to waste! I love refereeing. Good players appreciate having a decent referee get them through the game unscathed; bad players, on the other hand, are not at all happy, because they keep getting pulled up for fouls, get cautioned (yellow cards) and have to pay fines. Great fun.

Heather and I made plans for a trip to Sydney, Australia in September 2007, to attend her nephew's wedding. I had only agreed to such a long trip with the proviso that we would visit China on the way. I'd been fascinated by China for a long time and combining it with the Australian trip saved us a ton of money. Note the accountant's rationale at work here.

We arrived in Beijing on September 11, and it lived up to all my expectations. The only somewhat unexpected thing was the overall friendliness, hospitality, and courtesy of the people. On the first night, it rained torrentially, and Wangfujing Street was turned into a river. What a sight, all these beautifully-dressed Chinese ladies running along, laughing aloud, completely unfazed, while trying to keep dry under inadequate bits of paper.

At Mutianyu, we achieved "Hero" status for having climbed the Great Wall. We also visited the Forbidden City, which is an experience that I would recommend to anyone. If you do go, make sure that you don't miss Beihai Park, just to the north, a favourite of the Imperial Princesses some centuries ago. They liked to go there for a bit of R&R and to enjoy a fabulous view of the Forbidden City.

It was in the park that we got a birds-eye view (pun intended) of why most Chinese people seem so relaxed. We saw a man walking his pigeon. Yes, a pigeon. Now, clearly, you cannot rush when walking a pigeon even if the pigeon is not on a leash; their legs are too short so you simply must slow down to the pigeon's pace. Every so often, the pigeon seemed to get tired and flew up onto the man's shoulder for a brief ride while he kept walking at the same measured pace. After a while, he would say something to the pigeon and it would fly off his shoulder and start walking again.

We must have watched that man and his pigeon for about twenty minutes. It was almost hypnotic, and it made us slow down and relax as well. Probably a good thing, as I had a little trouble climbing the Great Wall and up to the Princess' relaxing place in Beihai Park, but over all it wasn't too bad.

On our third day in China, we flew down to Xi'an for the day to see the Terracacotta Army. Domestic flights in China are an excellent value with their new aircraft and efficient, attractive staff. The soldiers were amazing, and though it looks like it will be a very long restoration job I think it will be worth it. It's difficult to comprehend the impact of those endless rows of individually sculpted soldiers unless you have seen them in person.

When we got back to Beijing, we visited the Hutongs, an ancient district in Beijing with narrow streets or alleys formed by lines of courtyard residences. Houses are set up in quadrangles, with shared bathroom facilities at the end of the street. Prior to Chairman

Mao's regime, one family owned a whole courtyard, but he decided that was way too much house for one family, and split them into four. Today, families have taken the opportunity to buy up the rest of the courtyard and return the houses to their former glory. We were privileged to be shown around some of them. We were a little concerned that our pedi-cab driver would not last the day given his obvious maturity and our combined weight, but our fears were groundless: he was obviously fitter than either of us, pedalling away happily as we relaxed in the back.

We climbed the Drum Tower where drums were pounded in ancient times to call the people to work as there were no clocks in people's homes back then. That climb proved a little difficult as it is 100 (count them!) steps. There was an ingenious water-driven clock which told the drummers the time of day. The drums were played while we were there. The sound from those 10-foot high drums was incredibly powerful. There is also a Bell Tower a few blocks away where bells were rung to send the workers home at the end of the work day.

Off to Oz

My brother-in-law Paul lives in a suburb of Sydney, Australia, and our first trip downtown was quite an event. We took a water bus down the river. What a lovely way to commute, no traffic woes at all. It's just like a normal bus with regular stops, except it's on the river.

Paul's home backs on to woodland (bush) and interestingly they are required to clear the undergrowth occasionally to avoid the very high risk of bush fires. Imagine that, right in Sydney's suburbs! It's great for walking, although Heather and I managed to get lost and ended up doing an unscheduled 10k hike.

We enjoyed a boat trip through the bay area in a tour boat operated by aboriginals. The guide told us quite a bit about the history of his people, and gave us an excellent demonstration of how to play the didgeridoo. The trick is breathing in and out through the nose while blowing through the instrument to make the unique musical sounds. We saw the same player performing on the quay back in Sydney later. He seemed to be quite the entrepreneur.

Something unique to the Sydney scene is the DIY BBQ/Restaurant/ Pub. We joined a bunch of Paul's friends at a place called The Oak, where you can select whatever meat or fish you want from the butcher's station, take it to a huge BBQ and cook it the way you like it. It's a great way to meet people. The guys stand around the BBQ, cooking meat and potatoes and drinking beer, while the ladies chat away at the table. Once the meat is cooked you just grab some of the vegetables provided and enjoy. We loved the concept and went to a couple of different spots during our stay. The wedding was a fun event with family and friends and took place in a beautiful garden setting. We were so glad we could be there to celebrate the happy occasion.

Home via Hong Kong

We headed back to see Dr. Dancey, who by now had all my test results, and a diagnosis. I had Pulmonary Fibrosis. He guided me carefully through the CT scan images, pointing out the various areas of scarring in my lungs. I do appreciate a doctor who is not afraid to give you complete information, one who does so in layman's terms. He quizzed me about possible causes. Had I ever worked in a coal mine or around asbestos? No. Had I ever been on a bird farm? Well, we had a budgie once. No, that wouldn't do it. Did I smoke? No, I'd stopped in 1983. That couldn't be it either then. Since there was no apparent cause, I had what was defined as Idiopathic Pulmonary Fibrosis (IPF). So, it was a disease of unknown origin, and therefore there was no treatment. That news was not very comforting at all.

Dr. Dancey kept up with all the latest developments and told me that the only "cure" available for my disease was a lung transplant. While I was nowhere near that stage yet, Toronto General Hospital Lung Transplant Unit liked to start monitoring patients early, as Pulmonary Fibrosis is unpredictable and things can deteriorate quickly.

He said he would arrange an appointment with Dr. Singer at Toronto General. He also indicated that he would be available in the interim should I have questions or concerns, which was reassuring. I could make an appointment or just drop by, and he would always see me if he was free.

At my next meeting with my family doctor, she strongly advised me to get a flu shot and a pneumonia shot as my lungs would be more vulnerable, and these viruses could be fatal. The pneumonia shot was good for ten years, but the flu shot was to be an annual affair. No problem; I had been getting the flu shot for some years anyway.

I moved on to my new life, facing all sorts of challenges that evolved over time. Some of these challenges had to be addressed personally, with support from family and friends, while others could only be overcome with the assistance of an arsenal of professionals and the resources at their disposal. Pulmonary Fibrosis is not a nice disease. You need, and should take, all the help you can get.

Chapter 3 **The First Year**

Western medicine does not have a monopoly on successful treatments for chronic diseases. My previous experience with Traditional Chinese Medicine (TCM) had been a positive experience. I had been treated for depression by Dr. Susan Sun and felt I benefited far more from TCM than from all the drugs and psychiatric counselling I had received over the years. I did some research on the Internet and found that the Chinese had reportedly had some success in controlling Pulmonary Fibrosis using their treatments.

Dr. Susan is an expert in all areas of TCM and after consulting with a former hospital colleague who did work in this area, I was prescribed a mix of various herbs, told to boil them, and inhale the fumes. I had to drink some herbal tea which I didn't enjoy, but Pulmonary Fibrosis patients will take anything that may help when there is no other treatment available. I soon got used to the taste.

Christmas 2007 was a bit subdued, as we considered a future that now included Pulmonary Fibrosis, and what that might mean to us all. We were determined not to let it take over our lives. Although we knew Heather's friend had died so quickly from it, I truly believed it could be beaten. I firmly believe that when we face a grim diagnosis that we should continue to enjoy life while educating ourselves on all aspects of the disease.

It was disappointing to discover the lack of information about Pulmonary Fibrosis and the low level of funding for research. Even in the U.S., there was only about $30 million a year being spent on research in spite of the very high death rate among those suffering from the disease. The number of deaths annually was the same as for breast cancer and prostate cancer, though there were far fewer people afflicted with Pulmonary Fibrosis. Research leads to effective treatment and cures, but it takes money, *lots* of money.

* * *

Dr. Dancey arranged for me to see the Lung Transplant Unit doctors at Toronto General Hospital (TGH), in January 2008. Dr Singer, as expected, told me I was not ready to be put on the list yet. I knew that, as I was still able to referee senior soccer without getting too winded. In fact, I felt pretty good. She explained the process that would occur as the disease progressed, including the transplant assessment procedure, and she let us know what would be required of us if I was ever put on the transplant list. She indicated that I was somewhat overweight to be operated on for a lung transplant, which I assured her would be remedied. Ironically, that turned out to be easier done than said.

I was assigned a transplant assessment coordinator (a registered nurse with special training in this area), who gave us a copy of the Lung Transplant Patient Manual, a large 170-page book containing everything you need to know but were afraid to ask. It is very comprehensive and covers all aspects of the program and then some.

As soon as we got home, we both read the manual cover to cover. The side effects of the drugs looked pretty formidable. Apparently, some people decide against a transplant after reading about the potential side effects. I felt that for me, the side effects were nowhere near as bad as described, and certainly they were no worse than death.

I was told to keep seeing Dr. Dancey, but I would also be having appointments at TGH every six months. That meant I saw a respirologist every two to three months, which was fine by me. Being closely monitored by experts couldn't be anything but good, even if there was nothing they could do about the disease yet.

The Canadian health system is world class if you have a serious illness. I know that's not always obvious, especially when you're seeking treatment for a minor health problem or have to endure hours waiting in emergency. But surely a health system should not be judged on how it deals with flu epidemics alone. It should be evaluated on the strength of its response to life-and-death situations. I have no complaints at all in that regard.

* * *

I am a chartered accountant and had quite a pleasant little tax practice with some great clients, many of them becoming good friends. The busiest time for my practice was from February to mid-July. After that it calmed down to a nice steady pace work with a comfortable lull until September. The busy season that year came and went much as usual.

I had been refereeing at The USA Cup in Minnesota for about 15 years. This was a fabulous, week-long, international youth soccer tournament, which was at one time the biggest in the world. My first time there was with my youngest son, Matthew, when his team from the Scarborough Soccer Club decided to participate.

There were over 700 teams that year with almost 13,000 soccer players attending. The opening ceremonies, which were organized Olympic-style, were really impressive. It's great to see that many kids interested in playing the "beautiful game." Matthew's team went on to win the grand finale, conducting themselves like real sportsmen throughout the tournament.

Over the years, I made many friends from every part of the world; teams and officials come from 22 countries. As one of 400 referees, meeting and working with officials from so many different countries is a real thrill. Soccer is a simple game with uncomplicated rules, but it still amazes me how we all manage to interpret them in very similar ways, no matter what language we speak or where we come from. Soccer truly brings the world together with no room for racism. Some things are simply universal, like a kid kicking a ball around.

In 2008 I decided to attend the tournament again as a referee. It was to be memorable, but not in a good way. I had a heart attack that put me out of action on Day 1.

I was assigned a middle on a 15-year-old boys' game. That's a super age to referee as they've developed some skills but are also discovering hormones, and you do need to keep on top of them. I had an English referee on one line and an American on the other. I wasn't feeling too great, so I told the Assessor (a Welshman), to hang around in case we needed him. If I had to bow out of the game part-way through, the English referee, who was named the senior assistant for that game, would take over and the Assessor could do his line.

I don't think he liked the idea of running a line because I looked over after about twenty minutes, and he'd disappeared. Later, he jokingly told me I failed the assessment. "How do you know?" I asked him, "You weren't there."

I managed to finish that game and was assistant on the next one, an under-13 boys' game, but I still wasn't feeling well and was not very impressive. Thirteen-year-olds were outrunning me!

On the way back to the headquarters I felt quite ill and had to stop and rest often, so I went to the dormitory and lay on my bed. I was only there for a few minutes when I felt bad enough to go to the first aid centre, which I knew was fully staffed with five doctors and a number of nurses. I staggered downstairs and was fortunate enough to run into Mike, one of the general helper volunteers and a really great guy, who drove me to the centre in his golf cart.

Well, they were quite thrilled to see me, as they were mostly dealing with mundane stuff like sprains, broken arms and legs and heat stroke and exhaustion. Now they've got a suspected heart attack and a chance to exercise more of their skills. The only problem was that the communication link between the angiogram machine and the local hospital wasn't working. Thankfully, the doctors were alert and decided that I probably was having a heart attack; they sent me to hospital by ambulance.

The paramedic in the ambulance asked me if I wanted to be taken to the local hospital or the one at Coon Rapids. (Don't you love the names of those mid-west U.S. towns? Somehow it conjures up visions of hundreds of gleeful raccoons shooting the falls.) If it was a heart attack then they would ship me to Coon Rapids anyway, whereas if they took me straight there I would save on ambulance fees. At $1,750 a pop, all I could say was "Coon Rapids, here I come!" I hope TD Insurance appreciates my stringent economy on their behalf.

Talking of which, I only bought the insurance the day before my flight. I have to say that this was forward thinking on my part and what excellent value it proved to be. Oddly enough, after the paperwork was completed and my friendly TD agent had assured me I was now covered in the U.S. I had facetiously remarked that I supposed I could now have a heart attack with impunity. Honestly, I did not intend to put it to the test. I won't be joking about that in future, I can assure you.

When I got into emergency, they did some tests and confirmed I was indeed having a heart attack. I was about to get an inkling of the differences between the Canadian and U.S. health systems. Bringing the cardiac surgeon in over the weekend meant he would have to be paid double time, so they would just monitor me and operate on Monday. Wait a minute, this was Saturday, isn't time of the essence when dealing with heart attacks?

I survived, and had a stent put in on the Monday, which was a pretty simple procedure to open up the clogged artery in the heart and improve the blood flow. I'd had two of these done previously in Canada where it was basically an overnight event. Go in, have the procedure and go home the next morning. At Coon Rapids, they kept me until Wednesday, and at $12,200 a night, who can blame them? Their health system is, after all, profit-driven.

I can't think why, but the tournament directors wouldn't let me referee any more games that week although I did look after the penalty shoot-outs in the playoffs, which was a bit of fun, and it gave me something to do. A couple of the first aid centre doctors saw me in uniform that day and asked what I was up to. When I told them I was working an under-19 boys' game at three o'clock they nearly had heart attacks themselves.

So much for trying to live life ignoring the pulmonary fibrosis. Something always happens to interfere with my best-laid plans.

* * *

My wife and I decided to take it a bit easier on the travel front in 2008 by staying closer to home. We love Quebec City, with its tremendous history: interesting bistros and restaurants, dinner or lunch cruises along the St. Lawrence, and friendly people. It also has the added benefit of being only a seven-hour drive away.

Although it was the Festival of New France, celebrating Quebec City's 400-year anniversary, we managed to get a room in a small boutique inn in the old city, just opposite Chateau Frontenac. Fortunately, it had an elevator as we were on the fourth floor. We walked all around the old walled city and along the boardwalk, a three- kilometre walk along the side of the cliffs and up to the Citadel, first built by Lord Dufferin.

The city is built on the cliffs on the side of the St. Lawrence River, so it tends to have a lot of downhill walks to the waterfront. Sadly, where there is downhill there must be uphill, and I really started to feel those climbs. I found I preferred walking the boardwalk from the Citadel side down rather than taking all those steps up. It did seem as if the Pulmonary Fibrosis was trying to get my attention. It was a gentle but unwelcome reminder that life as I knew it was changing.

The city puts on a full calendar of events and performances during their various festivals, and this time was no exception. On one of our downhill walks we came across a group of young Quebecois playing drums in the street. Their whole show was intense, chock-full of energy and the heart-stopping (not really) rhythm of various types of drums. They were a highlight of our visit.

Stay-at-home trips within Canada can rival anything abroad, espe-cially if you approach it with an open mind. It can really cultivate an awareness of our vast country's history, and can give you an appreciation for the role played by whichever part you are visiting, especially if you're ready to meet the local people and celebrate their unique culture and traditions.

* * *

Breathing Should Never Be Hard Work

Towards the end of December, I caught a cold I couldn't shake off. As we went into a new year it went into my chest. I believe now that this progressed the Pulmonary Fibrosis as I seemed to still be shorter of breath even after the cold had gone away. A little more of my lungs were rendered useless.

We had to start facing up to the reality of pulmonary fibrosis and its unpredictability.

Chapter 4   Bucket List Time

As the Pulmonary Fibrosis progressed (seems funny to use that word in regards to an illness) I gradually lost my appetite. This wasn't all bad as I needed to lose some weight in order to qualify for a lung transplant. I am 6 foot 1 and 235 pounds (185 cm and 106 kg). By the time I got the transplant I was down to less than 165 pounds (74kg). Needless to say, I do *not* recommend the PF Diet to anyone.

We all have a bucket list of sorts and I decided I'd better take a look at mine and then go ahead and do some of the things I'd always wanted to do. It wasn't that I'd lost faith in my ability to beat this thing, I was still planning on going for the full eighteen years. I had even appropriated Winston Churchill's "...never surrender. Never!" wartime vow.

I had thoroughly enjoyed China and wanted to see a lot more of it. Heather didn't want to use up her limited vacation days going again, so I was quite prepared to go by myself. When I was younger, I often went off to Italy on my own, relying on the friendly locals to join me in a good time, and I already knew the same would be true in China.

Heather did not share my enthusiasm for my solo trek to a country where I didn't speak the language and where the medical system was a complete unknown, especially as it related to my condition. Much to her relief my friend Clyde decided to join me. I suspect she was probably still a bit worried, knowing the dynamic duo's tendency to get into trouble when left to their own devices.

Dr. Susan suggested I might enjoy Yunnan province, in the far southwest part of China. It is quite mountainous and is known as the Province of Eternal Spring due to its pleasant climate. I found a tour company based in Xi'an who would provide us with guides and drivers as well as arrange for our internal flights to Xi'an and Beijing. We would start in Kunming, the capital of Yunnan, and finish in the fabled Shangri La, close to the border with Tibet. A quick visit to Google Earth told me that Shangri La was at an altitude of 3900 metres (12,800 feet). Hmm... would that be an issue?

When I asked Dr. Dancey if being at that altitude would be a problem he didn't exactly tear his hair out, but he came close. He clutched his head with both hands, sighed, and said "Nobody in your position has *ever* asked me that."

Knowing how determined I was, he sent me to Dr. Singer at TGH for an altitude test that confirmed I was OK at 2,590 metres (8,500 feet), so I was "allowed" to go. I was to find out later that there is a considerable difference between sitting down being tested on a machine in Toronto and galloping around up in the Himalayas. Live and learn.

We arrived in Kunming after a one-night stay in Hong Kong and were met by our guide. Vivian was a 23-year-old charmer who spoke excellent English and had a vast knowledge of Yunnan, Kunming, and its history. All the guides on our trip had university degrees and were obviously very proud of their country and its many cultural attractions. Vivian was tiny; compared to Clyde and me she looked very small indeed. She turned out to be one of the nicest guides of the whole trip.

We were taken outside the city to the Stone Forest, which is a huge natural area where the rocks have been worn down over the ages so that they now appear as trees standing separately in a forest. Some of them looked like animals and other figures. We saw a sleeping lion, mother and child, elephants and many other shapes designed and shaped by winds and erosion over the years.

While walking around the Stone Forest I encountered a very large water buffalo. These are quite common throughout Yunnan, where they are used in farming, and it's not uncommon to see them wandering down the highway, sometimes accompanied by the farmer.

I asked Clyde to take a photo and went to stand by this beast with the big horns. Clyde and Vivian got quite alarmed and told me to back off, as they were known to be dangerous. It looked pretty friendly to me, so I got my picture. I've never been that close to such an animal before. This is one of the reasons why I love travel.

Vivian suggested we see a dance and music production that was being shown in the main theatre in Kunming, called *The Legends of Yunnan*. The lead dancer was one of China's most famous dancers. She was born in Dali, also in Yunnan Province, and she is renowned for her White Peacock dance. The White Peacock is the Province's symbol for happiness and good luck. The show was absolutely magnificent, with stirring music and colourful costumes.

As China gets wealthier there are more and more cars in major cities, causing a lot of traffic problems for which they appear to have been ill-prepared. They make the roads work for them rather than relying on normal driving rules and traffic signals. Going the wrong way on a one-way street seems to be acceptable, provided the other drivers know what you are doing. Somehow in the midst of the chaos, they just make it work.

I had been to China before and knew about the traffic. I told Clyde that I was going to take him up to the nearest major intersection (a couple of hundred metres away) to watch the traffic. He was a bit reluctant but I convinced him it would be fun. The walk uphill was a little hard on me so I had to walk slowly. "Chinese drivers are allowed to turn right on a red light" I said. "Watch when they turn right on a red. They don't look left first."

"Why not ?" asked Clyde.

"I suppose it's because they might see something coming." I answered.

He thought it was hilarious that they indeed didn't look left, they just *went,* relying on other drivers to move over. The three-lane section of road soon became four lanes, as obviously three were totally insufficient. The poor traffic control officer who tried to stop traffic to allow pedestrians to use the crosswalk dared only stick his sign out to stop the traffic lane nearest to him. Beyond that, pedestrians were on their own. Crossing the road in China is *not* for the faint of heart.

Clyde wondered why a local vendor didn't set up a couple of tables and sell beer to the tourists who would happily sit and watch the traffic for an hour or so. Traffic as a spectator sport, who'd have thought it?

We were put on a flight to Dali, and spent two days there with a new guide showing us the various sights and sounds in that ancient city. Nice girl, but the odd thing was she repeatedly referred to herself as "a beautiful princess looking after the two foreign visitors."

Our next destination was Lijiang, where we met our new guide, Andy. Lijiang is the only ancient Chinese city without a wall. Apparently, the Chinese word for a wall, when placed next to the name of the city founder, did not make for a complementary joint name. Who knew they had naming rights back then?

It's a beautiful city with three mountain streams flowing through it. We stayed in the old part of the city where no traffic is allowed. We spent a lot of time at restaurants sitting beside these streams, sampling local beer (notice a trend here?) and eating barbequed yak meat. Yak meat is very tasty if cooked properly, but is very tough otherwise.

One evening we watched five Chinese workmen cutting an old rowboat in half to decorate the side of the riverbank at the restaurant. I don't think any dozen municipal workers anywhere in the world could have been more ineffective, though they did get the job done eventually. Clyde and I still marvel about this rather wonderful work ethic and the effort involved. No doubt it makes for full employment.

It was in Lijiang that we both contracted a nasty case of the runs. We were convinced we had contracted it from eating in a restaurant that was not overly-concerned with hygiene. This problem dogged us all around China and made seeking out western-style washrooms a fairly constant imperative. Most washrooms in China are based on squatting over a hole in the floor which presented some difficulties for us, especially with me and my breathing issues and Clyde with his arthritis. Be glad you've been spared the visuals.

Lijiang is at a slightly higher altitude than Kunming, 2,900 metres (9,500 feet) versus 1,900 metres (6,200 feet). The altitude tolerance test I had taken back in Toronto was really designed for air travel (airlines keep the cabin pressure at a level of 8,500 feet). I just wasn't prepared for the reality of walking around at that altitude and I started to find it increasingly difficult to breathe comfortably. The fact that our driver had a habit of parking as far from our destinations as he could get didn't help matters.

Andy had us walking all over Lijiang at a brisk pace, even after I asked him to source some oxygen bottles for me. Eventually I got more direct with him and told him I was stopping for a rest and a beer. He seemed amazed, obviously believing that it was a waste of my precious time in China.

He still hadn't gotten the message when we took a side trip to an ancient village a few miles away. Cars are not allowed in the village, and after we'd parked and walked towards the village I was faced with a long steep hill. "Are we going up there?" I asked.

"Yes," replied Andy.

"Not going to happen."

Just then some other tourists went by on mules. Light bulb moment! Clyde asked Andy where we could get them and off they went, leaving me sitting on a little wall enjoying the passing scene, always fun, especially in a foreign country. While I sat there, a lady came out to get water from the outside tap. I asked if I could take her picture, but she politely declined.

Clyde and Andy returned with our two trusty steeds, Andy was going to walk. Clyde had got on the first one and the poor thing sagged visibly under the weight. Clyde's feet were almost touching the ground, and the owner was rightly concerned for his animal's survival; he wanted to substitute a bigger one at an increased price. Clyde made his feelings clear about that using some time-honoured Anglo-Saxon expressions. The owner apparently understood the tone, if not the words, because the price stayed the same.

Clambering up into the saddle left me quite breathless, but these mules were a godsend as we not only toured the village but went out into the surrounding countryside, herding cattle on the way. I'm afraid I had scant sympathy for Andy having to walk the extra miles. I had to stage another rebellion when we went to visit the first bend of the Yangtze River, a very important development in history of China. This time I refused to walk back uphill and told him to bring the van down to me. The altitude was really getting to me.

We visited Tiger Leaping Gorge on the way to Shangri La. Legend has it that the gorge, the highest in the world, got its name when a tiger that was being hunted by locals leapt across the gorge and escaped. Even though there was a large rock in the middle of the Yangtze at this point it was still quite a leap. A few entrepreneurial types were offering rides down to the foot of the gorge on chairs carried by two men using poles slung over their shoulders. It was an amazing sight as these men ran down the slope carrying their burdens. I really wanted to try it but Clyde was worried they would drop me, so I gave it a miss. Shame really, I wish I had done it.

We picked up our new guide, a young Tibetan lady, for our trip to Shangri La, which was about 30 km from the border. She was great fun, only 22, but she had a "Life Plan." She told us that Tibetan girls were allowed to take three husbands and she planned to do so. "Everyone has affairs, so I may as well take three husbands, then I don't need to have an affair."

Flawless logic, even Heather might agree.

Shangri La was just too much for me. I couldn't handle the altitude. There's a reason it's called "the roof of the world." Clyde went touring a local park and Buddhist monastery and I lay on my hotel room bed. The only oxygen available came in small canisters, which could only really be used for emergency purposes. I did get up for lunch in the old city for a typical Tibetan meal. The funny thing was that we got french fries as part of the meal. I am convinced they were cooked in yak fat as they were the tastiest fries I have had since I was a kid back in London, England, when chips were cooked in beef drippings.

The driver (a new one, but obviously trained at the same school) parked as far away as he could, so again I had to get him to bring the van to me. I wasn't taking any chances.

The following morning, on the way to the airport to go back to Kunming, we passed herds of domesticated yaks and I was instantly reminded of those mouth-watering fries.

I was not allowed to take the oxygen canisters on board the plane, so Clyde and I finished them off in the airport lounge with Clyde playing the fool and pretending he was intoxicated. The locals and a couple of tourists seemed bemused by his antics.

Breathing was much easier back in Kunming, where we spent another day visiting a beautiful park before flying to Xi'an so that Clyde could see the Terracotta Soldiers.

While we were in Xi'an our guide took us on a tour of the wall surrounding the city. The hard part was climbing the 120 steps to the top. The wall is high, but it is also extremely wide, about 15-18 metres (50-60 feet). We capped off our visit with another live show; they certainly know how to stage spectacular events here.

On to Beijing and The Great Wall. Our guide in Beijing was more mature than the Yunnan guides and was a bit of a hippie in floppy hats and wild skirts and blouses, and we really liked her a lot.

The visit to the Great Wall at Mutianyu was a lot harder for me than it had been on my previous trip. The steep hill up to the Wall was a greater challenge and being stopped and heckled by vendors was an opportunity to rest for a while and recover my breath. We didn't buy anything on the way up but Clyde promised he would stop on the way back down. I did make it but I was too exhausted to walk along the top of it and even Clyde didn't go far. It was worth the climb, though, as the view is almost as magnificent as the wall itself.

I am now a "Hero of the Great Wall" twice over!

When we got back down, Clyde learned all about the tenacity of Chinese vendors. The lady he had fobbed off earlier spotted him and grabbed his arm. She wasn't about to let go until he went into her shop. Picture a 90 pound (40.5 kg) tiny Chinese woman herding a 235 pound (105.75 kg) Newfoundlander into her shop and making him buy T-Shirts for his grandkids. Surrender and buy, buddy. Resistance is futile.

* * *

I still had no real appetite and at the rate I was going I wasn't too worried about achieving the proper Body Mass Index (<30) specified for transplant patients. Our hotel in Beijing had a magnificent buffet dinner with all sorts of fish and shellfish dishes, lamb, Kobe beef, etc. Clyde went for the buffet (Newfoundlanders love their fish) while I decided I might just be able to manage some Sushi. It took me almost ten minutes to get through one piece, which was a source of great amusement to Clyde. I gave up after three pieces and settled for a beer. Did I mention that Chinese beer is very good? The Germans taught them how to brew the stuff in the early 20th century, building a brewery in Tsingtao, just east of Beijing.

* * *

I do have one regret about our China trip. Chinese students will seize any opportunity to talk to foreigners in order to practice their English. We were walking back to our hotel one afternoon when one of these students joined us and asked if she could buy us a coffee and have a chat. Clyde wasn't feeling well so I made our excuses and we went on our way. I feel that I let her down. I should have been more thoughtful and made a greater effort to be accommodating.

We made our way back to Canada via Hong Kong. I had thoroughly enjoyed ticking off the first item on my Bucket list and I was grateful to Clyde for joining me and making the trip even more fun.

* * *

One of the symptoms of pulmonary fibrosis is a dry, hacking cough, and I had starting getting it with a vengeance. It can be quite painful to the point of throwing up. There is no reason for the coughing other than to satisfy the cough reflex, but it is very real to us. There is not much to be done about it although prednisone does help some people. Unfortunately, weight gain is one of the side effects. Not so good when they want you to lose weight for the transplant.

In 2009, the leading news story was the H1N1 influenza bug, or "Hini," as I called it. The mainstream news media made it into a huge deal. There is nothing like a good health scare to sell newspapers and they made the most of it. In the end, everyone who had a sniffle or cough was looked upon as a social pariah. Enter Typhoid Bob

It was the worst of times to be afflicted with a cough, and I was subjected to many worried looks and unkind comments. One fellow diner turned and told me my coughing was annoying him while he was eating. I tried to explain that I was not at all contagious, but he didn't want to hear it, he just wanted to eat his dinner in peace. I managed to refrain from suggesting he move to another table (he had, after all, sat there after we had been seated for quite some time, and must have heard me coughing before he sat down). On a number of occasions, both in Canada and in England, people pointedly got up and moved away. The irony is that *I* was probably at more risk from *them* than they were from me. I don't suppose I can altogether blame them, but it did hurt a little because I felt so helpless. It was something I had absolutely no control over. Just another unsettling side effect of Pulmonary Fibrosis, one not described in any of the websites from around the world.

I also noticed I had become sensitive to various smells. Caring ladies wanted to give me hugs, which I usually do enjoy, except that perfume made me cough even more. When Heather was cooking, even with the windows wide open, I had to retreat to another room and shut the doors, as cooking odours set me off. Barbecuing was of course out of the question.

My respirologist prescribed a type of puffer that he thought might help settle the cough, but to no avail. He decided to put me on 50 milligrams of prednisone, which is quite a high dosage. This did help with the cough, and while I got a "moon face" as a side effect, I didn't seem to put on weight. Maybe the lack of appetite spawned by the Pulmonary Fibrosis offset the weight gain effect of the prednisone. At last, some balance in my life.

* * *

2009 was the 25th anniversary of the USA Cup. A group of us (Canadian and English men and women) decided we would participate one more time in the hope that the organizers might do something extra to help the referees enjoy it more. We felt they had been taking advantage of us. All referees paid their own travel expenses, and it was costly to fly in from distant countries only to not be allocated enough games to cover those costs, never mind the additional expenses for room and board.

Well, all we got was a cheap T-shirt. Whoopee. No change there, then.

I must acknowledge that they were very good to me in recognizing my health limitations. This actually caused a bit of good-natured jealousy from my peers, as I got very easy but profitable games. Referees at this tournament are paid based on their grade, not on the type of games they officiate. I was still a grade 5 referee in the U.S., which is equivalent to a State referee, so I was paid $35 per middle and $27 per line (assistant referee). Game times range from 25-minute halves on a small (half) field for younger players age 9-12, to 45-minute halves on a full field for the 13-18 year-olds.

There is obviously a lot of running for the older age groups whereas for the under-11s and younger it's mainly walking.

I was assigned four or five "baby" games every day; all middles, and all paying $35. My friends got two or three games a day, lines and middles, and earned much less for considerably more running. I took a lot of ribbing, but I accepted it with good grace and suggested they were not capable of officiating at my level. This was validated when Dennis, an English friend of mine, was assigned a "little 'uns" game on the next pitch, and I had to advise him at half-time that it was dangerous to run while refereeing these games; you might tread on a small player.

In spite of the fact that these were all walking games, I was still truly out of breath after each one of them.

* * *

After I got back from the USA Cup, I learned that I was going to be assessed to evaluate my suitability for a lung transplant. It's important to understand that this is the first stage in maybe, just *maybe*, getting a lung transplant, and therefore a shot at life: quite an exciting development if you have Pulmonary Fibrosis. It's not like you have any other option.

The assessment is a weeklong affair with many tests, as well as counselling sessions with doctors, anaesthetists, dieticians, surgeons and social workers. Many of the appointments started early in morning and went on until quite late. Late was okay, but early was a bit more problematic, so we stayed at a downtown hotel which gave a reduced rate for TGH patients who were going through extensive testing over long periods.

I had CT scans checking my heart and lungs, X-rays and blood tests checking arterial blood gases. I had pulmonary function tests and a six-minute walk test. Then they gave me a test with an oximeter to test my oxygen saturation and a nuclear medicine test to determine which lung was doing the work required to keep me alive. This last one determines whether you need one or two lungs. Then there were a number of tests to make sure the heart was strong enough to withstand such a long and difficult operation. These included an angiogram, Thallium Persantine scan, ECG and exercise tests. The drugs you take after a transplant can deplete your calcium, so I also had a bone density scan.

This was an exhausting week, but all of it was necessary for me to get on "the list." It also gives the complete picture on your health.

The social worker questioned me on various lifestyle issues, pre-sumably to see if I was going to look after the lungs I might be given. I had no problem with this as it is the greatest gift anyone can ever receive. She caught me out with one question. Do I drink alcohol? Yes. How much? Two beers a day. At this stage, all the other doctors who have ever asked this question are satisfied with the answer. Not her. "Would that be pints or bottles?", she asked. That's the price you pay for having an English accent, I guess.

I seemed to have passed all the tests, thank goodness, but I wasn't on the transplant list yet.

* * *

I like to play golf even though I'm not very good at it. I think the lowest handicap I ever reached was 23. That's what comes of taking up the game late in life. However, it is an enjoyable (if sometimes frustrating) game. The only thing that brings you back every week is that fantastic drive on the 18th hole. With the right foursome, it can also be a very social game.

As the Pulmonary Fibrosis progressed (there's that funny word again!) I found it more and more difficult getting 'round the course. Even though I always took a cart, it was still necessary to climb on to the tee blocks, walk onto the greens and, in my case, to venture into the trees looking for my lost golf balls. Eventually I gave up looking for them and just dropped a ball on the fairway. I rarely got to hit off the tee first as that honour is left to the player with the lowest score on the previous hole. On the odd occasion when I did earn the honour, I could not take advantage of it because after climbing on to the tee (even a low one, a couple of feet high), I was left breathless, and in need of a rest before trying to swing a club.

My friends were very gracious about all this and waited patiently for me to get my breath back and continue playing. Friends are very important for anyone going through Pulmonary Fibrosis as they will support you through those tougher times.

* * *

Back to the bucket list(s), since this one was on Heather's list too. She had always wanted to visit Scotland, and I wanted to see the Edinburgh Tattoo. I love the sound of the pipes and drums, as it is such stirring music. It must be my Scottish blood. I know it seems strange that, being British, we had never done these things together, though I had at least visited Scotland in my youth. Then again, many Canadians have not visited parts of this great land, though I must admit, Canada is a *bit* bigger than the UK.

We decided to go in time for Heather's 60th birthday on August 8th, which was also the day the Tattoo started. Coincidentally, it was also the 60th anniversary of the Tattoo. Didn't I do well? I had to get lucky sometime.

Edinburgh is Scotland's capital, and it is a beautiful city. There is the Old Town, which includes the castle and the many ancient buildings and churches that grew up around it, and then there's the New Town, which was constructed in the 18th century, to house the rapidly growing population. Those who moved to the New Town were more affluent, leaving the poorer folk behind to endure the noise, poor sanitation, overcrowding and disease. The Old Town and castle were protected by the Nor Loch until it was drained to create Princes Street in the New Town. You can see the topography from the ramparts of the Castle

The Parliament of Scotland was in the Old Town until the Act of Union in 1707 moved Scottish government to England. The new Scottish Parliament is now back in the Old Town but the new purpose-built buildings are not nearly as attractive as the much older surrounding buildings, including the Palace of Holyroodhouse. Originally founded as an Abbey in 1128, it is just across the way and is the official residence of the British monarch in Scotland. It has served as the main residence of Scottish monarchs since the 15th century and the Queen spends one week here at the beginning of each summer to conduct state business.

While in Edinburgh, we stayed in a very nice bed and breakfast (B&B) which was within walking distance of the castle and the Old Town. We did walk in to town one day and back out on another occasion, but generally we took the bus as it was getting a little harder each day for me to handle long walks. Edinburgh is quite hilly with long, gradual hills that are quite taxing. Given our advanced years (over 60), we were eligible for very cheap daily bus passes, something to remember if you visit that wonderful country.

We decided to go for a tour of the castle on Friday, before the Tattoo, not only to scout out the event venue but also to see this magnificent place. It is built on a volcanic plug which gives it a sort of ominous look as the plug is black rock. It also means constant climbing to get to the top of the castle and visit the various attractions. My breathing was still getting worse, so I was very glad that transport was provided so that those requiring assistance can start their tour at the top and work their way down. This was a really thoughtful service which was provided completely free of charge. Very generous of the Scots!

We enjoyed touring this great castle, including viewing the Scottish Crown Jewels; who knows, they may be used again if Scotland decides to go it alone one day. There are wonderful views from the top, and it is easy to see where the Nor Loch was, now covered by the New Town. At one o'clock, the big gun was fired off. This is a large field gun at the top of the castle, facing east, and it is fired each day to let the town folk know the correct time. Be warned: it's quite a loud explosion.

We meandered down to the lower courtyard, taking in all the places to see, and looked up to where we would be sitting that evening at the Tattoo. It looked a bit of a climb for me.

As it was Heather's 60th birthday, we decided to find a nice place for dinner. After, all it's not every day one reaches such a milestone. Birthdays with zeros and fives are special.

We should have made a reservation, especially as it was the first day of the Tattoo.

Heather enjoyed her gourmet birthday meal in a 16th century covered alleyway just down the street from the castle gates. We found a modest sandwich shop in this very old part of Edinburgh, with bistro tables outside. It sold wine as well, so it wasn't a total loss, and she managed to see the humorous side of it. It's probably safe to say that she will always remember her extravagant 60th birthday dinner.

We returned in the evening for the Tattoo. It's quite a climb up the Royal Mile to get to the castle gates, so we joined all the other people needing extra time to get up there. We congregated in a little churchyard, and once all the musician's buses had passed by, we were allowed to proceed up the hill ahead of all the other visitors. It must have looked like a pilgrimage of the afflicted heading off for a miracle cure. Once inside the gates, we had to climb up about 30 or 40 stairs to our seats. That was hard, as I was getting more and more short of breath by now. Anyway, we settled in and were treated to a truly impressive and stirring show by various musical groups from around the world, including troupes from China, Holland, England, Africa and Canada.

The British Army put on a very moving tribute to the allied troops who were fighting in Afghanistan, and the Royal Air Force did a low-level fly-by. A fighter jet screaming overhead at an altitude of less than 60 metres is pretty impressive.

The show culminated in a lone piper playing from the ramparts of the castle opposite where we were sitting. The power of this music was amazing and almost eerie, and the whole performance was enough to bring a tear to the eye. Everyone should experience it.

There are many interesting stories from Edinburgh's colourful past. One of the best loved stories is that of Greyfriars Bobby, a little Skye terrier whose master (Auld Jock) died back in the late 19th century. For the remaining 11 years of Bobby's life, he went each day and sat by his master's grave at Greyfriars Church. When he died the faithful "wee dug" was buried in the graveyard next to his master. You can visit the grave sites and enjoy a pint and some excellent haggis at the pub next door, Bobby's monument is right outside. Give him a pat from me as you go by.

The next day we rented a car and started a tour of the Highlands. Heather decided she didn't want to try driving a standard shift on the left-hand side of the road, so I was the driver. I think she just wanted to enjoy the scenery and I don't blame her.

The first day we drove up to Inverness, and visited the site of the Battle of Culloden. The English won that one, and there is an excellent museum with detailed descriptions of events during the battle. We strolled around the battlefield which is set up with small flags to show the positions of both armies and the individual clans. It was a vicious fight, but the Highlanders were outnumbered and poorly armed. I'm always rooting for the underdog so my Scottish side won out on this one.

We carried on to Dingwall, a small town across the Cromarty Firth. This is where Tulloch Castle stands, the ancient seat of the Clan Davidson, built in the 12th century. This fine castle, not much bigger than a country mansion, is now a hotel and boasts four-poster beds in rooms with walls that are three feet thick. It is a beautiful place to stay, although the lack of elevators made it a bit difficult to get to our room on the third floor.

Supposedly, the castle is haunted by a female ghost known as the "Green Lady." We took the ghost tour one evening, and later I stayed behind for a nightcap with the bartender who conducted the tour while Heather went up to bed. Heather will tell that story as she was the one who got "haunted" that evening:

"We enjoyed a lovely evening with the ghost expert from the hotel. She took us on a tour of the castle and then proceeded to tell us the story of the ghost. The Davidson family owned the castle from 1762 to the 1900s. Many years ago, the young daughter of the then-owner of the castle was horrified to discover her father engaged in "hanky panky" with one of the chambermaids. She ran off in horror, only to fall down the stairs and break her neck. Her father died under mysterious circumstances quite some time later. A family portrait of Caroline Davidson and her children, including the tragic Elizabeth, hangs in the Great Hall. The master of the house is conspicuous by his absence, although there is a space behind Elizabeth, where he would have stood. Reputedly, he was painted out of the picture after the tragedy. Caroline, the famous "Green Lady" still walks the castle mourning her losses.

Our guide told us there had been many strange happenings reported by staff and guests since the castle became a hotel, especially in the room where the unseemly behaviour had taken place. We found out it was the room next to ours!

As Robert said, he went for a nightcap with our guide (he does like a little cognac now and then) and I proceeded up to our room. I turned the key in the lock and just as I opened the door, *all* of the lights went out! *Wow,* I thought, *I'm getting a visit from the ghost, how exciting!* So there I stood, but alas, no apparition appeared, just a maintenance man muttering, "fuses blown." How disappointing! Oh well, maybe next time."

* * *

Before we left we were treated to a climb up to the watchtower which provided a magnificent view of the surrounding highland countryside. These climbs were really starting to get to me, but this one was worth it.

We travelled on to Dornoch, which is only about 112 km from John o' Groats, the most northerly part of mainland Britain. This was another super castle hotel, but this one boasted the luxury of an elevator. Granted, it was just about big enough for one person plus a suitcase, always presuming the suitcase was balanced on your head. Nonetheless, it was a boon for this weary traveller. Across the street was the ancient 11th century Cathedral, and not far from town was Dunrobin Castle, which was the ancestral seat of the

Duke of Sutherland. It is a magnificent place, well worth a visit. It includes a lot of history about the Argyll and Sutherland Highlanders, a famous regiment which can trace its origins back to a volunteer cavalry regiment raised by the Duchess of Sutherland in 1779.

One of the most beautiful parts of Scotland is Glencoe on the Western coast. We drove along Loch Ness (without catching even a glimpse of "Nessie,"). We admired the whole area around Glencoe, stopping for lunch in a wonderful local pub/restaurant, and we passed Ben Nevis, the highest peak in Britain. It was absolutely fabulous scenery. Now we had seen the deepest loch (Loch Ness), and we had seen the highest peak.

Our next stop was Stirling, which is the site of two historic battles where the Scots defeated the English to win independence; the Battle of Stirling Bridge (1297) under William Wallace and the battle of Bannockburn (1314) under Robert the Bruce. Our hotel backed onto the site of the battle of Bannockburn and a huge equestrian statue of Robert the Bruce stands guard over the battlefield. It is quite a different feeling to walk where all those brave men died.

We could see the site of the battle of Stirling Bridge from the Wallace Monument. It contains William Wallace's sword, which is a giant 64-inch claymore. It was a 160-stair climb to see it, so I was unable to get to it. Heather made the climb and gave me a full report with accompanying photograph, but I would like to go back and take a look for myself one day.

Stirling Castle is the regimental headquarters of the Argyll and Sutherland Highlanders and dominates the City of Stirling. Another climb. I was beginning to think Scotland might get the better of me yet. Fortunately, it was not as big a climb as Edinburgh Castle because this time there was no complimentary limo ride available. Scottish castles can be formidable places, and Stirling Castle certainly fits that description. We were surprised by the sudden appearance of a pipe and drum band marching through the castle grounds; It was an unexpected treat. The castle has a gift shop staffed and run by the regiment, where I picked up a very smart *skean dhu* (dagger) with the Davidson Crest on the scabbard.

I was starting to feel the effects of my Pulmonary Fibrosis with all the climbing up and down hills and steps. All too soon it was time to go home.

We started on our return journey to Edinburgh, stopping on the way to see the Falkirk Wheel, an engineering masterpiece which moves boats through a lock on a wheel mechanism. This mechanism uses less power to move two boats and all that water than it takes to boil a kettle of water. We had lunch in the small town of Linlithgow. It's claim to fame is Linlithgow Palace, the birthplace of The Stewarts and the ill-fated Mary, Queen of Scots.

Scotland is a beautiful country; it is rich in history and is populated by some of the friendliest people in the world. I want to go back there again one day when I can see more of the sights without having to worry about a lack of breath.

We stopped off to visit family in England on the way back, as we had to connect through London's Heathrow Airport. Even though my mother was almost 90 at the time and not in the best of health herself, it was obvious to her that there was something wrong with me, although we had all decided to keep the details of my health problems from her. The rest of the family were fussing around me. I think they were afraid I was about to expire on them there and then. It was nice to see them all, though.

* * *

By now I was really feeling the lack of oxygen, so that was the end of any more bucket list traveling.

Chapter 5 **The Foundation**

There was still nowhere on the Internet for Canadians to go to research Pulmonary Fibrosis or, more importantly, to get some support. There was an excellent US site, but for obvious reasons much of the information was not applicable outside their borders. We needed a dedicated Canadian site for IPF patients. We decided to establish our own foundation to provide support to those suffering from Pulmonary Fibrosis and to raise much-needed research funds.

In early August, just before our trip to Scotland, I took out a letters patent for the Canadian Pulmonary Fibrosis Foundation (CPFF) and completed the necessary applications to ensure the Canada Revenue Agency would approve us as a Canadian Registered Charity so we could issue tax receipts for donations. It's a complex and time-consuming process, so being a Chartered Accountant made the task a lot easier and saved substantial professional fees.

After we got back from Scotland I contacted Canada Revenue to check on the progress. The first agent I spoke to suggested that it could be nine months before the application was processed. I told him I could be dead before then. He chuckled, but I was deadly serious. I eventually spoke to a more senior agent who managed to get the application approved by late October.

We were in business. Now to get the word out, though we had no idea how to go about it. Fortunately, my youngest son Matthew had completed his Masters in Sports Management in Europe, and in the course of his studies had met a lot of young people with awesome and diverse skills sets, including expertise in building web sites and designing logos. He was working as a brand marketing manager at Adidas in Germany, and he called on his international band of talented friends to collaborate in building a fine website, with a superb logo that defines Pulmonary Fibrosis very well. My contribution to the process was the slogan: "Breathing Should Never Be Hard Work." The words were heartfelt, as by now it was *very* hard work for me.

Some friends who ran their own charitable foundations contributed their knowledge and expertise. One commented that she admired my courage in starting a new charity. I now realize why she said what she did. It is quite demanding and involves a tremendous amount of work; but we also feel a lot of satisfaction when we are actually able to provide useful support to so many people. We have met some wonderful people, all of them very brave as they deal with the disease and the uncertainties of its relentless progression.

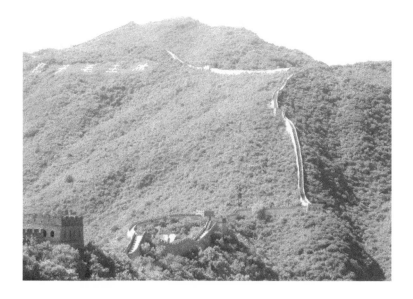

The Great Wall Of China. This was my second visit in May 2009 on one of my "Bucket List" trips. The views from here are magnificent, and it is a wonder that China was ever able to be invaded through these mountains.

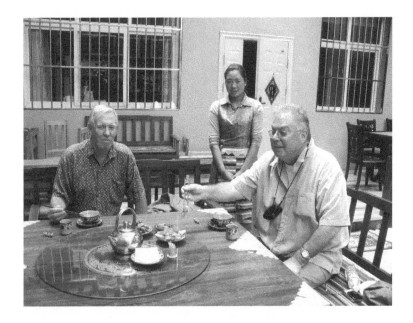

Clyde and I at lunch in Shangri La about 18 miles from the Tibetan border. The fries with this meal were delicious and I managed to get them down even with my loss of appetite.

After lunch I went back to my hotel bed. 12,800 feet up in the mountains was too high for me.

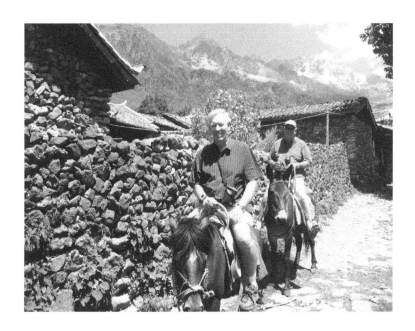

Riding the mules in Lijiang. Our guide, Andy, had to be persuaded to help hire these beasts so that I could go up the long steep hill. We got small revenge as we went extra miles into the countryside and Andy had to walk along beside us.

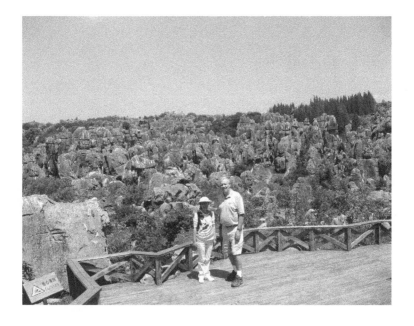

Me with Vivian, our Kunming guide in the Stone Forest. She was a delightful young woman and probably our best guide in Yunnan Province, China.

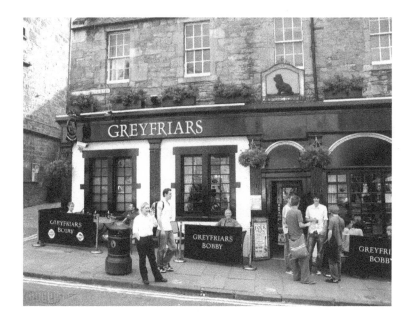

If you look closely, you can just see me sitting outside Greyfriars Bobby pub in Edinburgh, Scotland.

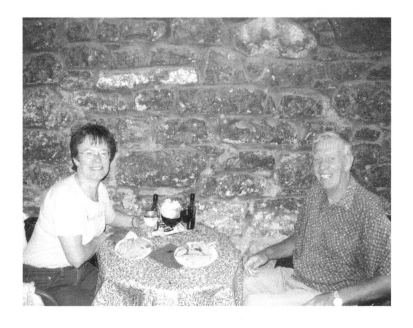

I don't think Heather will ever forget her 60th birthday dinner in an alley in Edinburgh. Sandwiches and little bottles of wine somehow seem a little more romantic in such an ancient setting.

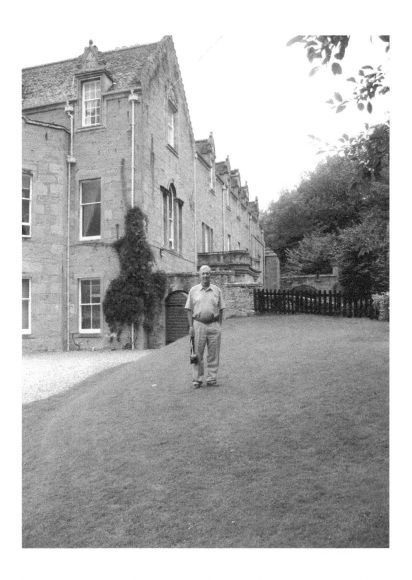

Me in the grounds of Tulloch Castle. Once the seat of the Davidson Clan, and now a very nice "haunted" hotel (unfortunately without an elevator). It was one of the best places I have ever stayed.

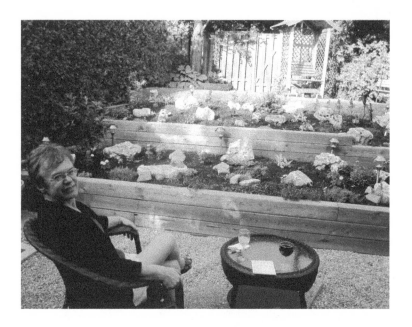

After my transplant I had so much energy. With the help of my son, Mark, and some friends, I built this rock garden less than four months after my operation. It could have been the heavy doses of steroids I was on, but I still enjoyed the work.

Heather enjoys sitting with a glass of wine out there.

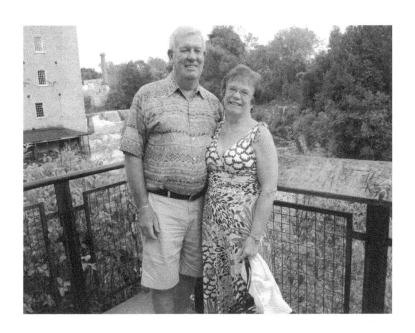

We took a little trip to Fergus, Ontario to see the Scottish Tattoo held there each year in August, seven months after my transplant. Our hotel room was right on the river, by the falls. It was very noisy but also very pretty. I was able to enjoy walks with Heather along the gorge.

Chapter 6   I'm Going into End Stage PF

Pulmonary fibrosis can smoulder away in the background, for an indeterminate time, without having much of an impact on your life. Then, without warning, something triggers it, and it gobbles up more of your lungs until breathing becomes extremely difficult. Mine was now doing just that!

As it worsens, more and more of the alveoli (the little sacs in the lungs which process oxygen) become, basically, lumps of scar tissue so the lungs cannot process the oxygen into the blood stream and filter out the waste carbon dioxide in the returning blood. The effect is a lot like suffocation. You constantly struggle to get oxygen into the body and everything you do takes a supreme effort. It becomes difficult to breathe and talk at the same time. Many times I had to stop talking and gasp for air. When the body is starved for oxygen it starts to divert the available oxygen to the organs that you need most to survive and so prevent respiratory arrest. As a result, the brain gets less oxygen and the memory starts to deteriorate. In addition the hands and feet get cold as the nice, warm, oxygenated blood doesn't get to the extremities. Not too good for cuddling the wife, but great for shock value. You can live without warm hands and feet and a good memory but you do need functioning major organs.

I like to go to the local pub, *The Duchess of Markham*, for "attitude adjustment hour". A group of us old guys sit around after work, have a couple of beers and generally solve all the world's problems. It's a mystery to me why the UN doesn't tap into these groups, they exist everywhere and are the repositories of so much accumulated wisdom that we could save the planet given half a chance. But I digress. In keeping with my "never surrender, Never!" mantra I vowed to keep meeting my friends no matter how hard it got. I refused to be defined by my illness.

In spite of all my precautions, I managed to catch a cold in early November. Even a cold can be a real killer when you have pulmonary fibrosis, especially if it gets into the lungs; it seems to cause the fibrosis to accelerate. That's one of the reasons we try to avoid being around people with any illness, particularly upper respiratory tract problems. The effect of this cold was pretty dramatic for me as my oxygen saturation (the amount of oxygen in the blood) went down to the mid-80s. Normal oxygen saturation is between 96 and 100 per cent. You can still do things at 85 to 90 per cent saturation, but for any strenuous activity supplementary oxygen may be required.

I was sent to the local hospital to be tested to see if I qualified for supplementary oxygen. The test is basically two six-minute walk tests, one with oxygen and one without. I easily qualified, so now I would have to carry around the oxygen I needed to stay alive. A strange concept when not so long ago I was fit enough to run around refereeing soccer games.

The oxygen arrived in four bottles, each about half the size of a scuba-diving air bottle. In order to get the most time out of each bottle they suggested the regulator be set at "demand" rather than "continuous." I tried that for about a week then decided it was just too difficult. I felt as if I had to suck the oxygen out of the bottle instead of just breathing normally so I changed the setting. I wondered whether they had received instructions to do this to save someone money.

The oxygen supplier delivered on weekdays only, except in case of emergency, in which case they would deliver on the weekend but at an additional cost. Each bottle lasted about 60 to 90 minutes and it soon became clear I would need more bottles. So now I had eight bottles, which lasted a week with careful management unless I got out of the chair and actually did something, in which case it was less. Next it was decided that I would be supplied with a refill system, a large tank about 100 centimetres high by 40 centimetres wide, which we placed in the corner of the dining room. So I was now set up with about a month's worth of oxygen. I'd had to increase the flow from four litres to six, although I never used it while sleeping. Dr Dancey told me I should use it at night but I didn't like the idea of going to bed with tubes stuck in my nose. I never had any problems. I think.

Later on, I was supplied with a concentrator - a machine that sat on the floor, plugged into an electrical supply and drew pure oxygen out of the air. It came with a fifty-foot breathing tube so I could walk around the house without lugging along a heavy tank. The only problem was that the tube, being made of clear plastic was almost invisible and Heather kept standing on it. Accidentally, she assured me. Seriously, not much fun at the time but we joke about it now. The other problem with this long tube dragging along behind is that it tends to get hung up on any obstacle in its path - and there were many - including chairs left all over the place for me to rest in. When I climbed the stairs to bed this was one of my worst fears. It took a tremendous effort just to screw up the courage to start the climb so any problem en route caused major frustration, anxiety and some-times tears. Shoes in the shoe tray were a constant irritant.

I was sent to Southlake Hospital in Newmarket for an angiogram to make sure my heart could take a lung transplant operation. I have been a mouth breather since I was very young, so when I wasn't getting enough oxygen by having the tubes stuck up my nose, I had the bright idea of putting them in my mouth. Problem solved. For some reason the nurses didn't agree, so every time one came by I quickly moved it to the required position. Happily I was only in there for the day.

Now, when I went to the pub I had to carry my oxygen in with me, use it and wait five minutes or so before I was able to enter the conversation. I thought this was bad, but it was to get worse. A lot worse.

* * *

Both my home and office had stairs,14 steps on the stairs at home and 20 at work. It was difficult enough at home but you would not believe the difference just six extra steps made. Getting up these office stairs every day was gruelling. Mercifully there was a landing half-way up both staircases so I could place a chair to collapse on. I took a three to five minute break on these chairs, even with oxygen, each time I made either climb. Week by week, it became more difficult. It was very easy to end up in tears as I climbed those stairs, gasping for breath.

Every event meant strong mental preparation to help survive the ever-increasing physical effort. You don't just get up from your chair and wander to the washroom, you sit there and build up the courage to move away from your comfort zone. I had to set up a line of chairs from wherever I was sitting to the washroom. I couldn't walk more than a couple of metres without the security of being able to stop for a rest. Imagine.

To add to my misery, it was around that time that I was put on an opiate for some reason that escapes me now. Thing is, opiates need to be accompanied by laxatives as they can cause constipation, sadly this fact seemed to have slipped everyone's mind, to my acute discomfort. Now washroom visits became an even greater challenge, so much so that I consciously avoided them, making the situation exponentially worse. My oxygen saturation sank to 61 per cent which was very painful. This was a huge problem, but it was also a salutary lesson. Discuss all possible drug side effects with your doctor and pharmacist. You really must take control of your own health. Panic time again.

* * *

By the middle of November I needed a wheelchair to get around the local mall, where they kindly lend you one for your shopping visit. I couldn't go anywhere else, unless it involved very little walking and offered lots of opportunities for resting. On the upside, I scored a disabled parking permit allowing me to park close to any entrance. At the mall I would wait in the car while Heather went to get a wheelchair and came back to get me and trundle me around. I did have a lot of fun engaging with passing toddlers. It gives you a different perspective being back down at that level and it was probably on a par with my mental capacity at the time.

When I wanted to go Christmas shopping it was Clyde to the rescue again. Friends are a great comfort when you have pulmonary fibrosis and I had some of the best. We spent a pleasant afternoon shopping and were careful to sit well away from the kitchen at lunch as cooking smells were now really bothering me. Now came the dreaded washroom visit. I couldn't put it off any longer. Clyde wheeled me in so I didn't have to walk far but standing there taking care of business almost caused me to pass out. Any exertion now was too much. Scary stuff.

This thing was getting worse and worse but I was determined not to give in to it. I ended up renting my own wheelchair. You can rent them by the month and I saw no reason why I should buy one. I wouldn't need it for long. I applied the same logic to the $11,000

Stairmaster. Why buy when you are soon not going to need it? The aftermarket is probably the same as for used cars, drive off the lot and lose 25 per cent of the value. Jump on a Stairmaster and you're immediately down $3,000. I was going to get a transplant, that's all there was to it.

Nice segue to the car. I drove a Chrysler 300M which was quite a decent car but it was seven years old and frankly I was bored with it. Clearly it was kismet because BMW had great deals on refurbished pre-owned cars and the prices were just right, with a great warranty package. Why not have another mid-life crisis and get a BMW? (My last mid-life crisis at 45 put me behind the wheel of a Jaguar XJS 12 cylinder beast but we won't go there.) After all, if worst came to worst, the life insurance proceeds would pay it off and then some and in the meantime I could have a little much-needed fun. So I bought the car, with a four year repayment schedule. Every cloud has a silver lining, or in this case, a dark blue one. After having fun with my sons, test driving several different models, I was the proud owner of an immaculate, low-mileage 3Series.

As it turned out, for the next six months the car was mostly driven by other people and I am still paying for it. In some respects I blame my friend, another Bob, who really encouraged (read pushed) me to buy it - and have all that fun - but honestly I don't regret a moment or a penny.

* * *

Christmas 2009, was probably one of the least enjoyable ever. I was now confined to a chair for the rest of the day after spending a gruelling couple of hours just getting up. We left the front door unlocked so visitors could just come straight in without me having to get up and stagger to the door and then totter back to my seat. After Christmas day sitting became much better as Heather had bought me a super reclining chair as a Christmas present. This worked out alright, though some of the delivery people probably thought it was weird when a disembodied voice shouted to come on in.

One day some very, very good friends, Bob and Brett, came to visit with their daughters, then aged 14 and 11. They came, not just to visit and offer support, but to make a donation to the Foundation. By the looks on the girls' faces I think they weren't sure I would survive their visit. Someone they were used to seeing as a sturdy, slightly overweight friend of their parents was now a shadow of his former self. An underweight guy with grey skin who might die at any time, maybe even while they were there. It must have been quite scary for kids that age. I didn't die and I truly appreciated their visit.

On December 23rd I found breathing so difficult I decided I had to brave the local hospital emergency room. Dr Dancey had given me his cell number and told me that if I had any problems over the holidays I was to have the hospital page him and he would be there. A truly caring man. I was admitted through emergency very quickly and sent for x- rays. When Dr Dancey arrived he confirmed the pulmonary fibrosis was worse and ordered another CT scan straight away.

There was nothing else that they could do for me so I was sent home with instructions to wait to hear from him.

* * *

Since the disease had progressed to the point that death was now a distinct possibility, Dr. Dancey, in whom I had complete trust, coura-geously raised the issue of advance directives, also known as living wills. We needed to think about our options in the event I could no longer breathe on my own, even with oxygen. If I was admitted to hospital with respiratory failure, I could be kept alive on a ventilator which would do my breathing for me. It would mean a tube down my throat for breathing, and a feeding tube. That used to mean that the patient could not be on any lung transplant list, but that was no longer the case. I would be fully conscious but unable to speak and would have to communicate by writing.

He suggested we discuss any instructions we might like to have in place for that eventuality. I asked how long I could be on a ventilator before I would be too weak for a transplant. Not very long, a few months maybe, but it would still be possible.

We went home and discussed this with both our sons. Matthew had come home from Germany so we could enjoy what we believed might be our last Christmas together. I felt that I would like to be kept going until such time as the doctors, in their best judgement, determined that a transplant was no longer possible under any circumstances. At that stage we would make our final goodbyes then have the tubes removed and accept the consequences. I believed I owed it to my family to buy as much time as possible to increase my chances of getting new lungs. I would hang on, using life support for as long as a transplant was still a viable option. No point going on beyond that.

Thankfully, Heather and the boys agreed with my position. There would be no fighting the inevitable and we would have the opportunity for a decent goodbye.

I drafted the instructions, signed them and had them witnessed:

Instructions For End Of Life Health Support

I ROBERT WILLIAM DAVIDSON of 47 Squire Bakers Lane Markham, Ontario being of sound mind, but not so sound body, do hereby give my wishes and instructions to my family and health professionals for the actions that I wish to be taken in managing my health in the event of respiratory failure requiring my admission to hospital and medical assistance for breathing and eating. I understand that I may be required to have assistance in breathing through a tube placed into my lungs, feeding through a tube to my stomach and other drastic interventions.

I wish these actions to be undertaken and continued so long as I remain eligible for a lung transplant. If, on the advice of Dr Lianne Singer of the Lung Transplant programme at Toronto General Hospital and Dr David Dancey of Markham, Ontario, my respirologist, together, I am definitely no longer eligible for a lung transplant due to medical issues that make such a transplant impossible I request that I be kept on the support system until such time as my family, Heather, my wife and Mark and Matthew, my sons can be at my side in the hospital.

Once I have had time with my family I wish it to be known that I do not wish to be left on support if there is no hope of recovery or lung transplant and nature must be left to take its course.

Signed
Robert Davidson

_____

Witness
A friend

_____

Date: January 5, 2011

* * *

We were having a quiet evening at home on December 28th when Dr. Dancey rang with what could be good news. He'd been pressing Dr Singer at Toronto General to follow up on an angiogram I had undergone in early December, as part of the process to see if my heart could take a serious operation, and then to get me listed. The cardiologist at TGH was still away for the holidays so no answer on that front, but Dr Singer had suggested that I stop taking my Plavix, which was an encouraging development. I had been taking Plavix since my first angioplasty in 2006 to thin the blood so that the heart didn't have such hard work pumping. Surgeons are not too keen on their patients bleeding too much, so when you are listed you must stop taking these drugs. It sounded like they might be willing to list me. Things were looking up. What a relief.

* * *

I had realized that I would not be able to properly service my clients in the upcoming tax season so I had started the process of looking for an associate to take over the day-to-day running of my practice. I was determined to find a person or group who would remain in the same location in Markham in order to provide an almost seamless transition for my clients. They needed to be chartered accountants as that was the level of professional expertise my clients expected, that's why they had come to me in the first place.

An acquaintance of the receptionist asked her if I would be selling my practice. If so, the chartered accounting firm he worked with would be interested. I met with them as well as a number of other chartered accountants and entered into an agreement with them effective January 1, 2010. In retrospect going with this group was not the best decision I could have made but at least my clients were looked after and didn't have to suddenly rush out to find new tax advisors at the worst possible time for them.

We're all allowed one mistake. These people did not look after my clients properly and as a result I lost a great deal of my practice, without compensation. I felt bad for those clients who were left struggling, and for myself as I contemplated a significant loss to my retirement plan.

A word to the wise. Every self-employed person should have both Long Term Disability Insurance and that wonderful product that wasn't around when I was starting out, Catastrophic Illness Insurance. These will certainly help carry you through such a stressful time in your life.

Chapter 7 **Transplant**

By January 2010, I was at rock-bottom health-wise, but I was still convinced that I would survive this thing. After all, I had a great family, super friends, and some of the best doctors in the world working with me.

Breathing was getting harder and harder, and the slightest activity sent me into hacking, coughing fits, leaving me gasping for breath even when plugged into my oxygen supply. Sometimes the coughing was so bad it caused me to throw up. However, I still insisted on visits to the pub for attitude adjustment hour; it just took me longer and longer to haul myself in there, resting every two or three yards. My friends were great. They understood that I could not begin talking until my oxygen saturation had moved into the 90 per cent range. I wore a wrist-mounted oxymeter to measure the saturation and remind myself of when to "stop and smell the roses." I'd bought it in advance of clambering about at high altitudes on my last trip to China, but now I used it all the time. Different mountain, more effort to climb.

Heather went to work about 7:30 in the morning, and I got up early too as I couldn't manage my morning routine without her help. It's really important morale-wise to keep things as normal as possible, and that includes maintaining your standards of personal hygiene and grooming. It is all too easy to gradually let yourself go due to the sheer effort involved, but if you let yourself go down that slippery slope, you are giving up and the disease wins. That is *definitely* not an option. I dreaded getting out of bed in the morning when faced with the pain of not being able to get sufficient breath to carry myself through my daily tasks. The loss of my independence was one of the hardest things to bear. I was totally dependent on Heather.

The morning's first challenge was the washroom visit, which often took two or three attempts. Before I could do anything, I had to get hooked up to the "umbilical cord" carrying my oxygen. So the routine became fixed. I'd get out of bed, take a couple of steps then turn and fall back onto the bed. Then I'd try again in a minute or so. Five minutes later, I'd give it another go, get scared and fall back into bed again. Eventually I was driven to succeed, motivated by my fear of the inevitable consequences of failure. The next stage was so much harder, showering.

Some years earlier my mother had been planning a visit from England. She was 83 at the time and had some health challenges, so we put a walk-in shower in the guest bathroom, complete with a built-in seat. Mum never made the trip (she's still alive though, at age 91) but now I was beyond grateful to reap the benefit of it.

When I felt ready, I would call Heather to come back upstairs so she could help with the next stage. While I lay on the bed she would turn on the shower, adjust the temperature for me and let me know when it was good to go. It's only about eight yards away but I had to get there in increments. I actually had to go past the shower to have a five-minute rest on the nearest bed in another room just to gather the energy to go for the shower. Hard to believe that such a short distance would be a major hike for me. I hardly ever managed to get there the first time around, turning back to lie on the bed again, but I am proud to say that for the most part I made it in three attempts.

Washing my hair was the hardest part, as I had to stand up, but it was all a huge effort. You need to understand that I couldn't wear my oxygen in the shower as I was a little afraid of getting water in the hose and inhaling it. Probably a silly idea but you get these peculiar notions, particularly when you feel very vulnerable.

As soon as I had finished washing, the oxygen supply went back in and the monumental struggle to get dry began, followed by the stagger back to the bed where I lay gasping for breath. This part really alarmed Heather as my stomach tended to hollow out and disappear into my backbone while my ribcage rose alarmingly towards the ceiling. She helped me finish getting dry and, after yet another rest, I would get dressed for the day.

With this, another major ordeal out of the way; I always felt so much better after a shower. I felt so lucky to have Heather by my side. I did try taking a bath once but getting in and out of the tub took more out of me, so the shower won out.

After a suitable rest, I made my way downstairs to our kitchen/family room and settled onto the couch. Heather then brought over a couple of the stools and set out the electric razor (a Christmas present from Mark), toothbrush, floss and toothpaste, along with two cups of water. With this setup I was able to complete the process while sitting down. This only took about forty five minutes.

Then I would plug the oxygen back in, and now I was set for the day. I would read the papers and watch TV, all the while dreading any need to go to the washroom as I still had vicious constipation. Thank goodness for the occasional nap.

Some days these arrangements took longer than others. On those days Heather would be late for work, but her employers and workmates were very understanding, enquiring about my health and how we were getting on under the circumstances.

I had no appetite, and solid food was very hard to get down, requiring a lot of chewing. A friend who is a sales representative with a natural food and vitamin company sourced a very large bottle of chocolate protein powder. Mixed with milk or water it was quite palatable and it went down easily, giving me the nourishment I needed.

I have been asked if, during this time, I ever considered the idea of death as a release from all of the pain and suffering. Although I often thought I was going to die at any moment, I never considered death to be a release, that would be surrender. I had to continue in the belief that I was going to somehow get back to normal; either I would get a lung transplant or some medical advance would arrive in time to save me. Also, I was not willing to put my family through the stress of dealing with my demise. You can endure. Giving up causes such hurt to those left behind.

* * *

When you go through the transplant assessment process at TGH, you are assigned a co-ordinator, a registered nurse, who organizes all aspects of patient care, including pre-transplant education and work-ups, scheduling appointments etc. Mine called in early January 2010 with an appointment to see Dr. Pierre, a thoracic surgeon. He would be the one doing my operation if it ever happened.

I wasn't on "the list" yet. He would make that decision at the meeting. As you can imagine, we went into it with a great deal of trepidation. He *could* say no.

When we met, Dr. Pierre was very pleasant and made us feel comfortable almost immediately. He went through the file and the notes from my assessment the previous July, particularly the notes from the anaesthetist, then discussed the operation in some detail. He did the usual work-up, took blood pressure readings, listened to my heart and lungs and a few additional things.

He outlined the transplant risks, including the fact that ten per cent of patients do not survive the operation. Seen in a more positive light: 90 per cent *do* survive. These are very acceptable odds when you consider that without a lung transplant the odds of dying are 100 per cent. When I went for an angiogram, I was warned that one in a thousand patients have serious issues; my cardiologist had done about 5,000 and hadn't had a single problem. I think they just like to cover all the bases. Damn statistics!

The lungs are a very fragile organ and are easily damaged, making some donor lungs unsuitable for transplant. They might have been previously exposed to environmental hazards, or they may have been damaged by the process of removing them from the body. Dr. Keshavjee, the Head of Research at Toronto General, had recently perfected a procedure whereby such damaged and otherwise unusable donor lungs could be repaired outside the body. This had the effect of increasing the potential lung supply by 25 per cent in one fell swoop. I was asked if I would be prepared to accept one of these lungs if they became available. He told us that, in his opinion, they were very often better than untreated lungs. I had no reservations at all and happily signed the consent form. I'd be only too grateful to take a "lung in a box."

In every operation of this nature there are other opportunities for gathering essential research material. In the course of the operation, the surgeons must cut through the sternum, and unavoidably some bone marrow leaks out. They asked for permission to harvest it, so they could use it for research. Otherwise it would only be re-absorbed into the body. This was another consent form gladly signed; I would do anything I could to facilitate research that may lead to a cure. A couple more research consents later and that was that. Now I just needed to sign the risk acceptance forms and I was on the list. Oh, happy day!

* * *

The transplant coordinator explained all the new things I would have to do, including applying for drug coverage with Trillium so that they would be assured I would be able to afford the costly drugs I would require for the rest of my post-transplant life. She also gave me the forms to get a pager at a special rate from Bell Mobility. They needed to be able to reach me 24/7. I also gave her all my other contact numbers. I had to stay within a two-and-a-half hour drive of TGH (lungs do not last long outside the body). If the On-Call Coordinator can't reach you within an hour they must select another recipient so you do not want to miss that call.

Now that I had been listed for transplant, I needed to get fit so that my health would be optimal, in order to eventually withstand the eight-hour-long operation. I know it seems odd but exercise does seem to help keep Pulmonary Fibrosis at bay. It probably has to do with the exercise keeping the remaining lung tissue as supple as possible.

The transplant unit doctors direct you to undertake a physical exercise program three times a week at the hospital. This continues until you receive the new lungs and for three months afterwards. I asked whether this could be done locally, but they wouldn't permit it as they had found that their program delivered superior results. Considering that any patient living outside the required radius has to uproot themselves and relocate for an unspecified time, it is a minor inconvenience for the rest of us to get there. I was glad in the end, as working alongside other transplant patients and those in post-operative rehab proved both inspiring and synergistic. These people displayed such humour and courage and we were all in the same boat, encouraging and supporting each other. After all, we were the only ones who truly knew how it felt to be in this position. We helped each other out through the many ups and downs.

My first session in the physiotherapy room was set for Wednesday, January 27, the following week. It would have been impossible for me to travel down to TGH alone as I couldn't get up to the 12th floor without assistance with my wheelchair. Heather was working and wouldn't be able to take me there every time, so I enlisted the help of friends. My first appointment was to receive an introduction to the various parts of the programme they had designed for me, so Heather took time off work to come to that one. It seemed a bit incongruous, bundling the wheelchair into the back of my nice, sporty BMW, but needs must be met, and so off we went.

Denise, the head physiotherapist, went through the exercise steps and equipment, then had me complete a full exercise routine which was shorter than what she would expect from me on a regular basis. I found it tough, but as it was my introduction I persevered, even though I did require a serious adjustment to my oxygen flow and its delivery method. I now had a mask over my face, taking oxygen when exerting myself. I was to bring this mask back to all my exercise sessions.

During the course of the session my oxygen saturation plummeted, and Denise was concerned enough to call in Susan, a nurse practitioner, to give me an examination. She immediately wrote out a new oxygen prescription for me, approving twelve litre flow. I was to present this to my home oxygen supplier who would then replace my tanks and regulators.

Denise suggested I start the full programme the next day, Thursday January 28. We had worked with my friends to put together a driver rota which went through to June. As luck would have it, on January 28th it was Clyde's turn.

I didn't expect him to stay with me during the full 75 minutes of my routine, but he decided he would, and I am glad he did. I got through all the warm up stuff, arm twirls and bends and stretches but it was incredibly difficult to walk on the treadmill, the first difficult part of the program. They wanted me to walk for 20 minutes as fast as I could. I couldn't do it. My oxygen saturation dropped to just above 70 per cent. Denise asked me to show her what I could do so I walked at half a mile an hour for just under five minutes then had to stop and sit down. I think this raised some alarms and I was told to cease and desist and come back Monday.

I was glad to get home and sink into my chair. Doing leg lifts on a recliner is not too difficult.

Friday, January 29th was a day like any other. I went through all the normal morning rituals (normal for *me,* that is) and at five o'clock I joined my friends at the pub for a couple of hours, then went back home for dinner and bedtime, as usual.

Everything changed on Saturday, January 30th at 12:23 a.m. when my bedside phone rang. I snapped awake to a voice asking, " Is this Robert Davidson?"

"Yes," I answered.

"This is the transplant unit at Toronto General, may I ask you some questions?"

"Yes."

"Do you have any infections?"

"No."

"Do you have a temperature?"

"No."

"We have been offered lungs; do you want them?"

Wow, I thought, *do I want them?* "Yes! I exclaimed.

"How soon can you get down here?"

"How about an hour and a half?" I answered.

It actually took a lot less time than that, which is amazing given the time it usually took me to get up and dressed. Never underestimate the power of the adrenaline rush. It can, given supreme motivation, overcome Pulmonary Fibrosis, albeit briefly.

I had been told that when we got the call I should not be the one to drive as I would be too excited and perhaps nervous. Really? Can't think why. Anyway, Heather drove. I'm still not sure who should have driven but it did give me a chance to make some telephone calls on the way.

I called Mark's cell phone first as he was sure to be out on a Friday night. Sure enough, he and his wife Alyshia were out with a group of their friends. I would have loved to have seen his face when I told him we were on the 407 on the way to TGH for a transplant. I told him he didn't need to come down as it could be hours before anything happened. We told him that we would keep him advised. I suppose it was a bit unrealistic to expect him not to go to the hospital, though. He told me afterwards that he was totally stunned, and just turned to Alyshia and said "We have to go, Dad's going in for a transplant!" They dropped everything and rushed straight to the hospital.

I then called Matthew in Germany, attempted to reassure him, told him I loved him and that Heather would call him again after the operation.

I also called my sisters, Anne and Carole, in England as I knew they would want to know, even if was only six in the morning their time.

At 1:40 a.m. we arrived in the emergency department as instructed, and were instantly admitted. Mark and Alyshia arrived shortly afterwards. A nurse came down from the transplant recovery room on the seventh floor and started preparing me for transfer to the third floor which is where the operating rooms are located. There was minimal paper work as it had mostly been completed back on January19, when I made it onto the list. While we were waiting we got talking with another patient who had been called in for a liver transplant. This was his second call down, the first liver had not been suitable. I hoped that wasn't going to happen to me. I found out later that he did get his new liver. Perhaps even from the same donor. We don't know.

Those two beers I had enjoyed earlier Friday evening and the subsequent chocolate protein drink were not going to be a problem, as we were not told until about seven a.m. on Saturday that the lungs were good, and that the operation would go ahead. They would take me to the operating room at 8:30 a.m.

Kisses and hugs went all round just before 8:30 a.m. and I was finally wheeled off to the operating room. I must confess to a little trepidation, more for my family's sake than my own. I don't think they were ready to be rid of me quite yet. For one thing they'd have to try and sell the BMW.

I was met outside the operating room by the anaesthetist who asked me again if I had ever shown any allergic reactions to anaesthetic to which I gave my standard negative answer. I don't react well to oxycocet though. No problem. We went into the room where I was met by a very pleasant operating room nurse who finished all the prep work, plugging me into oxygen and an IV, all the while chatting away, putting me at ease and telling me how brilliant the surgeons were.

I don't remember much after that. Actually, I remembered nothing at all until I woke up in the intensive care unit (ICU). After a lung transplant the patient passes through two ICUs. In the first one you are closely monitored, with a nurse for each patient. Then there is the second, the step-down ICU, where one nurse looks after two patients. After that it is down to the general ward where specially-trained transplant care nurses look after numerous patients.

All the while, Heather was waiting in the lounge with Mark and Alyshia, although she did eventually convince them to go home and take care of their little dog. She would call them when there was any news. Mark told me afterwards that they had seen a man walking by in the glass corridor opposite them, carrying an organ case, and they wondered whether it contained my lungs.

It must have taken a lot of courage for Heather to sit there all alone for so long, not knowing whether I was alive or dead. She is a brave woman and I doubt I could have done it with the same stoicism had our positions been reversed.

She told me later that the room phone kept ringing and it wasn't until a passing doctor poked his head in the door and said, "That's for you, you know," that she picked it up. It was the medical team reporting that the operation had gone well and that I was being transferred to the M/S ICU. I can only imagine how she felt at that moment.

The ICU was actually quite entertaining. The drugs they had given me, both during the operation and afterwards for pain control, were very strong and produced vivid hallucinations. Of course, I didn't know they were hallucinations, as they were very real to me. The first one, which was quite persistent, concerned a very loud argument between a police officer and a driver who was accused of being drunk. When asked why they had not stopped on the Gardiner Expressway when hailed by the police the driver's wife responded that she wanted to get to Toronto General as her husband had a serious lung problem. The police then asked why they had changed seats after stopping outside the hospital she advised them it was because she wanted her husband on the hospital side. I personally didn't think they had a chance, particularly when the police came back the next day with more questions. I commented to the ICU nurse that they were very loud down the hall.

"Who?" she asked.

"Those police with the drunk driver."

She just smiled, obviously used to delirious patients.

Heather came in to visit the day after the operation with a big smile on her face and, while she was there, they decided I could breathe on my own and would take out the ET tube that was deep in my throat. I signalled that I wanted to say something so they got a notepad and pencil. I wanted them to know that my last experience with this procedure had ended with me throwing up. Apparently they were used to that, so it was no problem. I didn't throw up and the tube came out beautifully.

The most amazing thing was the breathing. It was incredible! In fact, it was almost unbelievable. It just started happening on its own. Instantly, with no effort, I was taking big deep breaths and I had no pain. It is the most glorious feeling after months of struggling for breath. The feeling was indescribable. My voice was a bit hoarse, but that would pass. We knew I was going to be alright now.

In the step-down unit the hallucinations were different. Now I had TV on the ceiling, although for some unknown reason I couldn't change channels. I could move it around on the ceiling to wherever I was comfortable watching it, but the programme was not that great and finding a new channel would have helped. Very accommodating hospital service, fine drugs!

On Tuesday morning, two days after surgery I was transferred to the seventh-floor ward for recovery; it was a nice ward with a private room and super nurses. Visiting hours were pretty much unlimited, and the only restriction was a veto on flowers. Yep, breathing in pollen probably is not a good idea after a lung transplant.

I still had constipation, so dignity went right out the window. Never mind, the nurses were very polite and caring. I also had two tubes coming out of each side of my chest to drain excess fluids into two quite large boxes that I had to carry everywhere, including the washroom. These tubes meant I couldn't shower so it was sponge baths in bed. We all had a lot of laughs during that process.

I was now a member of a very exclusive club. Since 1983 there have only been about 1,500 lung transplants in Canada, and I had now joined their ranks.

Chapter 8 **Recovery**

Hospitalization is expensive so they want to move you on out as soon as possible. My rehab started almost immediately, with a visit from a physiotherapist on Tuesday afternoon. Did I feel up to some exercise? Absolutely. We hooked my "suitcases" (the chest draining boxes) to the side of a large walker, and off we went for a walk around the ward. The ward had a corridor that went 'round a central nurse's station, once around was 100 metres. After about 250 metres, she suggested maybe we should slow down. I was enjoying it way too much to stop anytime soon. I continued to do this circuit as often as possible, with or without the physiotherapist. It accomplished a couple of things: I got much-needed exercise and I met a whole bunch of nice people on my travels. I was doing about six circuits at a time, sometimes twice a day. Oxygen saturation never went below 98 per cent. Fantastic!

I met another lung transplant patient whose operation had taken place a week before and she told me I was quite an inspiration as she watched me gallop around the ward. I'd never thought of myself as a role model before, but I found I rather liked the idea.

Food, glorious food. Remember, I hadn't eaten properly for months, and suddenly I was hungry again. In fact, I was ravenous. Maybe it was the drugs, but I ate everything they gave me, even Mac and Cheese, which I detest. I ate everything they would give me. Strange how even banana bread with raspberry jam and fake butter can seem like a gourmet treat under certain circumstances.

I never did grasp the logic behind the dessert choices. My blood sugar was tested twice daily, as diabetes is a real concern after a transplant. Yet my tasty meal invariably included a fruit cup, butter tarts, or something similar. Why did they keep giving us these sugary desserts? I got a noncommittal response to my query so I ate them all and enjoyed every bite though I did learn quite quickly that it was best not to eat grapes right before a blood sugar test.

* * *

Toronto General is a teaching hospital, so doctor's visits tended to be quite social events, with up to five or six doctors crowding into the room. The senior doctor always asked permission for the juniors to be included and I always agreed. I figured that I might need those doctors one day. Some of them were from overseas and had come to TGH to study under the best; we also had student nurses from overseas. We have every reason to be proud of having such a world-class facility available to us. It saved my life.

You never knew which doctor was going to visit and order yet another test, but a visit from a thoracic surgeon was often a very good thing. They made the decisions about removing things like stitches, staples and, most importantly, drainage tubes. I really looked forward to those visits.

I had one complaint and that was related to the bed. Susan, the nurse practitioner, came to visit one day and I blamed the bed for giving me really bad back pains. She told me that they had spent a small fortune getting the best beds money could buy. Of course, I came to realize that it wasn't the beds at all. My chest had been cut open through all of the muscles from one side to the other and my sternum (breastbone) was held together with staples. What a whiner! It stands to reason that I would experience a backache.

I wasn't sleeping that well, so I was glad I had the little TV to watch in the middle of the night. The nurses wouldn't give me more sleeping pills at night, but they would give me painkillers if I asked for them. Some nights, even if I wasn't in pain, I would ask for one just to help me get back to sleep. You can only take so much HGTV. You'd think all that renovating and decorating would have tired me out, but it didn't happen.

I had friends and family visiting every day, including my son Matthew who decided he couldn't keep getting long distance reports in Germany, so he came back just to make sure no one was keeping information from him, as did my sister Anne, from England. I guess the speed of my recovery just seemed too good to be true. But it was a fact. I was the poster boy for TGH. I must admit, I had trouble understanding it myself. I put it down to the excellent care I received and the quality of the lungs my donor had given me. Those who visited could not believe the dramatic change. I was literally a new man, no longer grey-skinned and gasping for breath.

My memory returned. It had really deteriorated when I had been oxygen-starved. Now I was able to make phone calls from memory. My hands and feet were no longer permanently cold. No more icy cuddles for Heather!

The soft stitches came out first, on the Thursday. A few days later one of the drainage tubes was whipped out by one of the thoracic surgeons. When he got to the end of the tube he carefully removed it and used the single stitch holding it in to tie up the hole left by the tube, which was about half an inch wide. The other three tubes would have to wait until they were satisfied that the fluids were the right colour and volume. We all make these fluids in the lung cavity and it just drains away, but after a major operation like mine it was necessary to wait for the lungs to properly fill the cavity so that they didn't collapse.

When they came to take out the staples I was a bit apprehensive, but it was not at all painful. The staples holding my sternum together would just stay there forever. I wonder if they make it easier should I ever need a bypass operation, sort of like a zipper.

I can picture it now: "Good morning, Mr Davidson. We're going to do a triple-bypass today. Do you have a zipper we can use? The Ministry of Health likes us to save tax payers' money wherever possible."

Ten days after admittance, they took another tube out, so I was getting closer to discharge. Two down, two to go.

The team at the transplant centre don't want all their hard work to be wasted so they have you watch videos about your future health care before you are discharged. There's a mini-seminar to learn about prescription drug handling, side-effects and proper administration of each drug. The pharmacist visits immediately before discharge to give you all the prescriptions and go through the specific side effects of each drug prescribed. I found the videos helpful, because I absolutely wanted to look after the huge gift I had been given: new lungs and a new chance at life. How could I possibly live with myself if, after some brave person had signed their donor card and given me those lungs, I had squandered that gift?

By now I was on a first-name basis with all the nurses, nursing assistants and janitorial staff, and we were having a lot of fun. I would get to see them all again in just over a year when I returned to that ward with an infection. They were a great bunch of people.

On the second Wednesday, two thoracic surgeons came in, looked at the boxes, had a quick chat, looked at me and said they were taking the tubes out and I would be discharged on the Thursday. Without further ado, out came the remaining tubes, a quick stitch to close the gap and I was free at last. No more "suitcases." Another first.

On Thursday I had to wait until the nurses came in and took my final blood tests, pilled me up, and took my blood pressure and temperature before I could get up. I was going home! I had breakfast, showered, and got dressed, and I was ready to go at 9:30 a.m. *Come on, Heather. Come on, pharmacist.*

Heather arrived at about ten o'clock and we waited for the pharmacist together. Time dragged on. They brought my lunch. Poor Heather, she had to go downstairs to the coffee shop.

At last, the pharmacist arrived. Did I have any questions? You bet:

Could I have beer and wine while taking these drugs? Yes, the occasional one was OK. In fact, she enjoyed them too. Phew!

Next and most important question. Could we go now? Not quite yet, the doc had to come by and sign my discharge paperwork.

We finally left at about 3:30 p.m. I was sad to leave everyone, but was happy to know I wouldn't be too far away if I had any problems in the future.

It was twenty-two days from listing to discharge. How fortunate was I?

On the way home, I was reminded that life does not always go that smoothly. Sometimes we find ourselves the butt of a cosmic joke. I'll let Heather tell the story as she was the one driving and it was all her fault anyway:

"So excited! I was actually driving down the DVP to pick Robert up from Toronto General. He was alive! I still couldn't believe everything that had happened, and so quickly. Robert had gone from someone who was "on his last legs" to this smiling, joking man who could actually breathe normally, like the rest of us. Certainly, a miracle had happened, thanks to the donor, the donor's family, and a group of amazing doctors. Anyway, back to this story: I was circling the underground parking at the hospital looking for a space and happened to clip the curb. Oops! I carried on to park the car regardless, so eager to get up to Robert's room for his 11 o'clock discharge.

There he was, ready to come home, still grinning from ear to ear. Much, much later, after all the formalities, we went to fetch the car. Naturally, Robert noticed the flat tire immediately. I was horrified. All I wanted to do was to get him home as quickly and safely as possible. I called CAA and eventually a tow truck arrived. The serviceman inspected the tire and said he would put some air in it and it would get us home no problem. Famous last words.

We were heading north on the DVP when we realized that we could feel the dreaded bumpiness of a flat tire! I pulled over and put on the hazard lights. So much for tow truck driver No.1 and his optimistic prediction of an uneventful drive to Markham.

Once again, CAA sent the tow truck. By this time, I was practically certifiable but Robert was still smiling. He was breathing, so he didn't seem to care about anything else! Suddenly a police car pulled in ahead of us. The policeman was very helpful and offered to pull in behind us as a safety precaution while we waited. By this time the traffic was backing up for no good reason, other than every other passing driver's need to rubberneck. The tow truck arrived and then went to back up into place in front of us at, which point the driver behind him leaned on his horn. Our guy waved blithely and there was an exchange of words! Honour satisfied, he inspected the tire and told us we needed to put the spare on. He would tow us to a gas station where he could safely change the tire for us. Relax, Heather. Salvation is nigh. We just might make it home by supper time at this rate.

The tow truck driver was very amiable and really interested in Robert's story. Not many people get to meet someone who has just had a double lung transplant. He considerately made us go in the gas station booth to keep warm while he changed the flat tire, inspected the others and put some more air in one. It was bitterly cold, so we appreciated his efforts immensely. We bought him a coffee, waved him off with thanks and we were on our way again. We did get home safely. Robert was tired but still beaming. Nothing mattered to him except this amazing feeling of being able to breathe without thinking about it. So, if you were on the DVP in the rush hour on February 12, please accept our apologies, it was the Davidson's who caused that traffic jam. Given all that we had recently been through, it seemed we'd gone from the sublime to the ridiculous in the same day."

* * *

The next day, I decided I would go to the pub, just to let everyone know I was OK. Matthew came along as chauffeur. As I walked into the pub, everyone turned around to check out the new arrival. When they saw it was me they stood up and burst into spontaneous applause. It was truly a heart-warming moment. They were happy to see me and I was so glad for myself and my family. I had a grin plastered on my face that took weeks to fade away. One friend even asked if I'd had had the grin put on by a plastic surgeon while I was getting my new lungs. It looked that permanent.

* * *

Some of the side effects of the transplant took me completely by surprise. My emotions suddenly seemed to be very close to the surface. A happy story in the newspaper or on television would set me off and I would be holding back the tears. When people were nice to me, or to anyone else, it had the same effect. I suppose that after a life devoted to looking out for No.1, this could be seen as a positive development. I still get overly emotional over little things to this day. Since I also noticed that I now had some difficulty parking, I wondered if perhaps my new lungs came from a member of the fairer sex. But apparently women are actually better at parking cars than men, so much for that theory. I don't care either way; they work *wonderfully*.

Other changes happened right out of the blue. My taste buds were different. I no longer felt like coffee in the morning and I didn't eat apples and oranges for breakfast anymore. I didn't like broccoli at all and some other former favourites were right off the menu as well. No more glasses of milk. I think perhaps I took on some of my donor's characteristics.

* * *

I was on pretty high doses of prednisone which is an immunosuppressant; it's also a steroid. I was like the Energizer Bunny. I could have climbed Mount Everest. This was quite helpful as I had started my three months of post-transplant physiotherapy at the hospital.

It was very similar to the programme set out for the pre-transplant, but this time I was expected to improve each time. I had no trouble at all but I did land myself in trouble one day. The hospital discharge instructions told us not to lift anything heavier than ten pounds. One of the exercises had me lifting a seven pound weight over the shoulder with one hand then repeating it with the other. Why not save time by having a seven pound weight in each hand and doing the exercises together. Made perfect sense to me. I figured that I was only lifting seven pounds but I was quickly reprimanded for lifting fourteen pounds and told to do it properly. Busted.

I was not allowed to drive for three months so it was back to relying on others to get to the hospital. We dug out the original rota and five of my friends took control of the scheduling. I really appreciated this as getting to TGH by GO Train and subway and back home by bus would have taken forever. Mind you, I think they all got a real charge out of driving the BMW I had bought back when I believed my days were numbered.

The pre-transplant folks have yellow cards to record their progress whereas the post-transplants have green cards. I had many of the former ask me how long I had been on the list. When I told them it had only been ten days they were amazed. I met some really great and truly courageous people at physiotherapy. Turning up three times a week to exercise while coping with increasing supplemental oxygen requirements while hoping for lungs to come available must be incredibly difficult. It's got to be extremely challenging staying positive under these circumstances.

It was at physiotherapy that I first met Melissa, a bubbly 30-year-old from PEI who had first been diagnosed at the age of 21 and was put on oxygen at age 26, just after giving birth to her son. She had been listed a little before me and had a terrific attitude. I was so very glad when she got her new lungs. She was called down three times and each time she was sent back home again as the lungs were not suitable. Most other people would have despaired, but not her; she had everything to live for. She finally got her new lungs in November 2010, four months after her first call down. More about Melissa later.

To me these are real heroes, people who carry on fighting a killer disease, waiting for new lungs, and never giving up hope.

* * *

For the first three months I had weekly blood tests, X-rays and pulmonary function tests which meant I made yet another bunch of new friends in the labs (I sometimes felt like a pin cushion). There are some real benefits to this transplant business!

Everything checked out. All was well. At three months I had the full assessment: bronchoscopy, blood, pulmonary function, X-rays, CT scan and a clinic appointment where the doctor grilled me about *everything* after reviewing the test results.

I would also have annual bone density tests as the anti-rejection drugs can cause osteoporosis, and a gastro-emptying test. I have no idea what that last one's about but you have to go with the flow. After all, they were clever enough to give me new lungs, so I figured that they must know what they are doing.

These full assessments were carried out every three months for the first year and then every six months in Year Two. They will be carrying out various tests monthly or annually for the rest of my life. I hope I have lots.

They definitely don't plan on losing a patient to something fixable.

Chapter 9 **Rejections and Infections**

The body views the transplanted lungs as a foreign body that is attacking the host, so it reacts accordingly and does what it is supposed to do. It tries to kick them out, leading to rejection. Organ transplant recipients must take a regimen of anti-rejection drugs to suppress this reaction. The drugs are very effective once the proper dosage and balance is achieved, but that requires a bit of experimentation to fine-tune it to the individual. Immune systems come in varying strengths; some react more strongly than others to the new organs.

There are three grades of rejection. Grade 1 can be treated by an adjustment to the anti-rejection drugs while Grade 2 is a little more serious, requiring more aggressive treatment. Grade 3 puts you back in hospital.

My first rejection was a Grade 2, within the first three months. I didn't feel any different and my daily pulmonary function test still showed my lungs were working at 116 per cent of what was predicted (I know 116% is impossible it is just their way of measuring expectations that results in these strange results. I was just doing better than expected) . The rejection was discovered after one of my regular bronchoscopies. I was having one every month and without them I might never have known my body was trying to reject the lungs.

The treatment to counteract the rejection is an intravenous dose of 900 milligrams of prednisone for three days in a row, followed by heavy doses of prednisone pills for four weeks, reducing by five milligrams a week until you are back to the normal dosage. After that there would be an adjustment to the anti-rejection drugs.

As I was still not allowed to drive, a very pleasant and friendly nurse came to the house to set up the IV. It was a bit of a nuisance wearing the intravenous needle for three days, but I managed without ripping it out of my arm.

The second rejection, also a Grade 2, happened a couple of months later. Again it was discovered during one of my monthly bronchoscopies, also going unnoticed by me and my daily pulmonary function test. Although the treatment was the same I was now able to drive, so I had to go to TGH to have the prednisone drips.

I found out about that one while walking along the street in July 2010, just after I had been to Southlake Hospital in Newmarket to have another stent inserted into one of my cardiac arteries. My cell phone rang and it was the hospital calling to let me know about the bronchoscopy results. They instructed me to come down to the hospital right away to get my treatments. Matthew was over from Germany again and had borrowed my car, so I had to call him and ask him to come back to Markham and get me down to TGH stat. I went for a haircut while I waited for him. This was a little bit of excitement for him on his short vacation in Canada.

My third rejection, also picked up through a bronchoscopy, was only Grade 1. At last we were getting somewhere. This one was dealt with through a change in medication. I was taken off Cyclosporine and put on a new drug called Prograf.

Unfortunately that last bronchoscopy also detected two serious infections. Normally there would have been no dire consequences, except that I was immuno-suppressed.

Cytomegalovirus (CMV) is a virus that can cause disease in different parts of the body. In lung transplant patients it can result in pneumonia, which of course can be fatal.

Most people are exposed to CMV in their lifetime, but typically only those with weakened immune systems become ill from that CMV infection. Usually it produces no symptoms, but very serious CMV infections can occur in people with weakened immune systems due to organ transplants, or those taking medicines that suppress the immune system.

Once you become infected, the virus is with you for life, but it's usually dormant. You rarely get a recurrence unless your immune system is suppressed. CMV infection in an immuno-compromised person can be life-threatening.

The CMV had reared its ugly head and was giving me an infection. The treatment is a very expensive drug: $3,200 per month for three months. I started on it immediately.

I had also contracted a fungal disease in my right lung which can also be very dangerous. The treatment for this was yet another costly drug at $3,400 a month. .

Thank goodness I had a drug plan.

These drugs interact with Prograf so I was placed on a lower dosage, five milligrams twice a day. There were no problems with this new drug at all. Unfortunately, drug reactions are usually dose-related, so I didn't find out about my reaction to it until I had completed the drug courses for the two infections (fungus and CMV). Once I had finished those drugs and the doctors had confirmed the infections had both been dealt with, they increased my Prograf to thirty milligrams twice a day.

At that level, I started feeling all the side effects, and I was also getting more infections. I was put on another drug for chronic infection, so now I was taking 42 pills a day. This seems to be my new status quo. Again, when I consider the alternative, I don't mind at all.

Some of the drug side effects are dizziness, occasional blurring of vision, lack of sleep, weight gain, hearing loss and fairly strong hand tremors. It can be quite a lot of fun trying to read while holding the reading material in my hands. I have, on occasion, gone to the doctors alarmed by some of these side effects. Once I am reassured they are not life-threatening I can get on with life knowing what I'm dealing with, although I must admit I preferred the Cyclosporine which caused me no side effects.

Like all immuno-suppressed people I get infections quite regularly; some of them I can I fight off on my own, and some require medications. I will continue to have these issues for the rest of my life, but that's okay with me as I now *have* a "rest of my life," for quite a long time. I just have to learn to avoid people with colds and flu, keep my hands clean all the time, and use a lot of common sense. It could be infinitely worse.

At the time of writing, the last rejection episode was eighteen months ago. During that time I was getting regular bronchoscopies and blood tests, so I am quite certain the rejection days are behind me now. They may return, but by then there will probably be new and improved treatments.

We are told to watch out for certain symptoms which are indications the body is trying to reject the lungs. The first time I thought I detected a problem I went to my local hospital emergency department. I explained the symptoms and that I had received a double lung transplant on January 30, 2010. Four hours later I was seen by a doctor. Had I actually been experiencing a rejection, those four hours could have been critical.

That experience taught me a lesson. Next time I went straight to emergency at TGH. I had recorded a temperature of 37.5 early in the morning and during the morning it had climbed to 39 degrees. While this may not sound like much, it is considered quite high risk for transplant patients. I was processed through emergency very quickly and was in the care of a doctor within an hour of arrival. They understood the potential problems following a lung transplant.

It turned out that I had pneumonitis, a very dangerous, and possibly life-threatening virus for lung transplant recipients. I spent a very pleasant five days renewing my friendships with the nursing staff on the 7th floor, most of whom remembered me from my previous stay. It was a bit miserable being in isolation, but they certainly sorted out the problem. They are such caring people, all of them with a great sense of humour.

Chapter 10   Galas, Golf and Fundraising

The Foundation had received some major start-up support from friends, but we still needed to come up with ways to raise more money in order to make meaningful research grants.

My daughter-in-law, Alyshia, and her mother, Maryann, had organized a Spring Gala to be held at a local banquet hall in Markham in April 2010. This was to be the Foundation's first major fundraiser, and we were holding it less than three months after my transplant. At this stage I was still not allowed to drive, so getting around to pick up donated auction items and raffle prizes was a challenge. Thank goodness all of the actual event planning was done by Alyshia and Maryann.

I had never realised how stressful it could be to run such an event and I was really impressed by all the work they did in selecting the venue, organizing the delicious meal, choosing the entertainment and hiring such a fantastic DJ.

The evening went extremely well and we were able to raise over $12,000, which I think was excellent for our first event. Everyone enjoyed themselves and promised to attend the event next year. The DJ Alyshia had chosen got the party started early on, and kept it going right to the end.

Although I was 63 at the time (though my lungs were only 28) I can't remember ever giving a major public speech. But, as the President of the Foundation I was expected to speak at our first event. It was easier than I thought, especially now that I could breathe again. I spoke for about ten minutes to a hushed crowd of over 200 people, many of whom had never met me before. Those strange new emotions I mentioned earlier came to the fore when I got to the parts about the people in pre-transplant physiotherapy, and my donor, but nobody seemed to mind.

I got the second standing ovation of my life, so I guess I did alright.

* * *

Our next event was a golf tournament which we held at Angus Glen Golf Club. I had been involved with another charity's golf tournament held there, so I knew they would help make it successful. It was a little expensive but I believe it was worth it. We had a lot of volunteers for this event and were given many excellent raffle prizes, but getting the players was very difficult, even though many friends were pushing ticket sales. I had lost most of my own network, having been out of circulation for a couple of years. We ended up with 91 paying players, nine short of our guaranteed 100. Not bad for our first attempt. The weather was miserable, cold, windy, and it rained for the first three holes. This didn't put a damper on things. Despite the weather, everyone said they had a good time and that it was a well-organized tournament. We still managed to raise over $10,000, so I was happy with the first annual CPFF golf tournament. As this was the final fundraiser of the year, we decided to make the presentation of our first grant at the dinner that evening.

I had contacted Dr. Chan at University Health Network (UHN) in Toronto to enquire about any IPF research projects currently underway which might require additional funding. He referred me to Dr. Ted Marras and Dr. Shane Shapera who promptly put together a funding request to cover the cost of a research study Dr. Shapera wanted to start, which would look into the relationship between Gastroesophageal Reflux Disease (GERD) and IPF. We approved this project as one we would like to fund, since it related directly to IPF research, and I had suffered from GERD for many years. I didn't know it at the time but $50,000 is considered a lot of money in the research community.

Doctors Marras and Shapera came to the golf dinner, accepted our cheque for $52,000, and made a very informative speech of thanks which included a review of GERD and IPF, scaring a large portion of their audience as they considered their own experiences vis-à-vis acid reflux.

We hadn't actually collected all the funds at the time, so I had to lend the Foundation $7,000 for a couple of weeks. It was worth it to get some research going.

* * *

We started getting donations from across the country, given to us by people who had lost a family member or friend to Pulmonary Fibrosis. It seemed like the web site was having some success in getting our name out there.

I was also receiving a lot of emails and telephone calls from people who had been diagnosed with IPF and didn't know what to do next or where to turn to for help. Although the stories were sometimes tragic, and always came from people who were scared and needed answers, I did appreciate these opportunities to help. After all, this was the very reason we had started the Foundation, to provide support to those who needed it and to pass on my own experiences. I started making a lot of new friends.

Almost all of the calls I received were from people who not only had been given the frightening diagnosis, but had also been given no hope, not even a referral to the lung transplant programmes where they lived. Many were advised they were too old, even if they were younger than I was at the time of my transplant.

It really reinforced how lucky I was with my respirologist and how inconsistent health care providers can be across the country.

* * *

My son, Matthew, had written to many of the groups who organize charity marathons across Canada enquiring about entering their events. He was sure that the fundraising opportunities would pay off without too much effort on my part.

In February 2011, just after my one-year medical assessment, I received an email from the Scotiabank coordinator of the Halifax Bluenose Marathon, being held the last weekend in May, asking if the Foundation was interested in entering the event. By complete coincidence I received a telephone call the next day from Tara. She was currently living in Toronto, completing her Masters at University of Toronto. Her father, who lived in Sydney, Nova Scotia, had recently been diagnosed with IPF. She had found our web site and wanted to volunteer to help, either by fundraising or in some other way.

I told her that I had only just been contacted by the Halifax marathon people and asked if by any chance her family ran. Serendipity or what? Her mother had completed a half-marathon the previous October and Tara was certain she and her family would want to get involved, so I went ahead and entered the Foundation in the event. What a momentous decision that proved to be! Tara's whole family worked tirelessly getting runners and sponsors. I decided to travel to Halifax for the event and walk the 10k event. Tara's family also did the 10k, including her father; her mother and one sister ran the whole way.

It turned out to be an amazing weekend. I drove out to Halifax as I had shirts and coffee mugs for the CPFF participants, stopping on the way to visit a lady in Nova Scotia who also had Pulmonary Fibrosis and wanted to meet "the man in the picture." My photo had appeared in an article in the Halifax newspaper about my participation only a year after my transplant.

I'd forgotten how hilly Halifax is. I couldn't find a downhill anywhere. I started off well, almost keeping up with the rest of them. Hey, someone has to bring up the rear and make sure no one's left behind! It fell to myself and a petite lady, under five feet tall, to bravely fulfill this function. It was a little disconcerting when she spotted her son, picked up the pace and left me in her dust.

After the event, in which I was soundly beaten by everyone, including Tara's father (who, remember, has IPF) we dropped into a nearby pub for some much-needed refreshment. Later on, we met up again for a very nice dinner. What a great bunch of people and what a nice family. By the way, we raised $11,000, an amazing achievement. I'm going back in 2012.

Our second entry into the Halifax Scotiabank Bluenose Marathon became part of our 40th wedding anniversary and my 65th birthday. Heather and I treated ourselves to a trip to Prague to celebrate the anniversary, an anniversary that two years previously we really didn't believe we would see.

Two days after returning to Canada we left for Halifax to take part in the 10k event on the May long weekend and to renew our acquaintance with our new Nova Scotia friends. Sheila, one of our organizers in Nova Scotia whose husband Peter has IPF, is quite competitive and was determined to beat me in sponsorships. As a result we raised over $14,000 on this occasion. And she did beat me, bless her heart. Once again I was beaten handily in the "race", this time by Heather who came in about 15 minutes ahead of me. I still finished the 10k, though.

* * *

I had been instructed not to travel by air for at least a year after my transplant, I'm not sure why, however, my mother's 90th birthday was on April 8th and Heather's father's was on the 5th. What better excuse to travel to England than a couple of 90th birthday parties? Also, my mother wanted to see for herself that I was okay. Both she and Heather's father were delighted to have us help celebrate their birthdays, and we had a lot of fun with family and friends. Of course I took the opportunity to hit up my family for sponsorship for the Halifax 10k, and Heather did the same with her relatives.

Matthew was still living in Nuremberg, so we took an additional week to visit him. He took us to see various sites, including Munich and Salzburg, Austria, which was a two-hour drive away (and was the home of Mozart). The castle in Salzburg is usually accessible by a funicular built in the early 19th century. Wouldn't you know? It was out of service during our visit. I was elated to be able to climb up over 240 steps to get us half-way up, followed by a long walk up a winding pathway to the castle at the top. Not bad after a double lung transplant.

* * *

We had planned the second Annual Gala for April 16, 2011 so although we enjoyed our trip to England and Germany, it probably wasn't the best of times to be away as we were busy trying to sell tickets. The timing was particularly bad as Maryanne had also planned a cruise at the same time. However, we did manage to have almost 180 people attend and still raised over $12,000.

I had organized a local Chinese dance studio to entertain us with a short recital. They actually did three of them in the end. The troupe was made up of kids from four to about twelve years of age, and they put on quite a show. The audience loved them.

I had been the speaker at the previous year's dinner and I didn't think they would be that interested in hearing from me again so I asked my new friend, Melissa, if she would like to speak. Remember Melissa from rehab? She had a six year-old son who at that time had never seen his Mummy without her oxygen line. I am happy to say that she seems to have been given lungs that function as well as mine do.

She was a little nervous about speaking to such a large group, but as soon as she realized they were on her side and hanging onto every word she said, she relaxed and told her story so powerfully that most of the audience were in tears. I suspect the remainder felt the same but were working hard to hold back their emotions.

* * *

The same Melissa emailed me one day with the news that the Team Transplant dragon boat team needed more paddlers, particularly men. She told me where to go for a Wednesday evening practice on Lake Ontario where I would see the team milling about. Strangely enough, it turned out she had broken her ankle, so she couldn't participate for the rest of the season.

The team is made up of people who were either organ transplant recipients, living donors, (mainly kidney) or people waiting for a transplant.

I paddled with the team for the balance of the 2011 season and thoroughly enjoyed the exercise. We entered the Barrie Festival but only managed to come in third. That's alright, there's room for improvement. I'll be doing it again next year.

Dragon boat racing is good fun and a fine workout for the heart and lungs (which I need to get in both cases), so I signed up again for 2012. Our first race was in Parry Sound, Ontario. We easily beat the opposition in the first two races but only managed 3rd in the last one. Once again we were short of paddlers, so we conscripted four young paddlers from the local dragon boat club. I think these 13 and 14-year-old athletes were quite intrigued to be paddling alongside all these folk with spare parts all over the place.

We did manage to win the Wellness Cup which was a side event between four boats manned by teams with health-related issues. All in all, it was a good day.

* * *

The local soccer league in Scarborough, a Toronto suburb, hosts an International soccer tournament in aid of Cystic Fibrosis Canada. The referees for this event donate their time and are the major sponsors of the tournament.

I was pleased to be able to participate as a referee again in July 2010 and used it to get more free publicity for the Foundation. I worked three games over the weekend and enjoyed every one. It was just like old times.

* * *

In September we held our second Golf tournament at Angus Glen. This time I decided to run a silent auction with items we had acquired or that had been donated.

Although the day was dry and sunny, it was still a bit chilly with a north wind. It did seem like we were making progress. Maybe in 2012 it would be warm and dry. Again, we didn't make our minimum number of golfers but everyone enjoyed the day and we had good raffle prizes and trophies, including trophies for men's and women's "Most Enjoyable Day," which went down well. I am not a fan of "Most Honest Golfer" trophies. It's supposed to be fun. We raised another $11,000.

In discussions with the UHN doctors as to where we should allocate the grant money, they suggested that with $50,000 available, we could fund a Research Fellowship. This meant we would provide sufficient funds for a fully-qualified and recently graduated doctor of Respirology to devote four days a week to research at the Interstitial Lung Disease unit at TGH. The fifth day would involve clinical work at the hospital. I thought this was a great way to get the most out of the money we had raised, and after dinner we were able to present a cheque for the full $50,000.

After I had made the presentation, I was delighted to receive, on behalf of the Canadian Pulmonary Fibrosis Foundation, The Upper Canada Medal presented by TGH for excellence in supporting health research.

The Upper Canada Medal was first struck to provide recognition of the distinguished service and bravery of the volunteers in the War of 1812. After the war the medals, which were made of gold, were melted down and the bullion used to establish The Toronto General Hospital. Seems very fitting somehow.

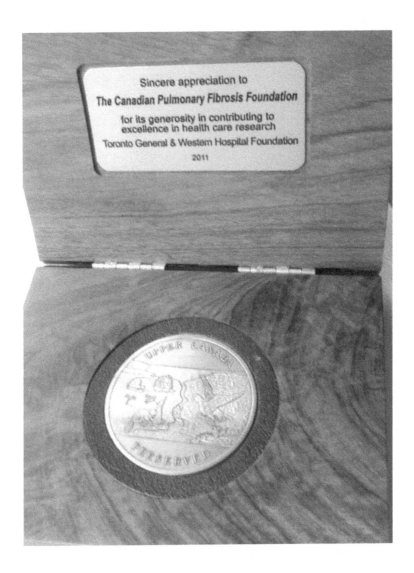

The medal states on one side "Presented by A Grateful Country" encircling the words "For Merit". We are very proud indeed to have been given this award.

Chapter 11   **The Future**

It's been over two years since I received my new lungs, and while I still take 42 pills a day and have to constantly guard against infections, I feel so good. I have celebrated three birthdays, including my 65th, that I would not have seen without the transplant. Every birthday is confirmation of the miracle I live every day. We have also had two more family Christmases, and more importantly, as I mentioned in the previous chapter, on May 27 of 2012, my wife and I celebrated our 40th wedding anniversary.

In July 2012, Mark and Alyshia presented us with our first grandchild, Alexis Ava. Just think, I may never have had that thrill to look forward to without so many events aligning so favourably.

I do feel different and I know that those around me cannot truly comprehend how I feel about having someone else's lungs giving me the breath of life. I am not sure I understand the whole thing myself. I am here only because someone else, someone who may have been a better person than me, decided to consider other people in the event of their own death, and then they did something about it. Every so often, when I am at the hospital for tests, I go to the physiotherapy room and chat with other lung transplant patients, just so I can talk with someone who is also walking around living with new lungs.

When I had my operation, 50 per cent of transplant patients survived for five years; today it is 55 per cent. Research is going on continually to improve survival rates, and researchers at TGH are conducting stem cell research which will trick the body into believing the lungs are not a foreign body. Researchers are also working on drugs to slow down or stop the scarring process. IPF patients would be quite happy to carry on with their lives knowing that the Pulmonary Fibrosis will not get any worse. We can live with a bit of scarring. Some of these drugs are already approved for use in Japan and Europe, but research goes on to further develop and improve therapies.

We will be having our third golf tournament in the Fall. Every day and every anniversary is a gift to be celebrated.

We will shortly be giving another $70,000 for a research fellowship at TGH. We are also seeking out a good use for another $20,000. That means grants totalling $192,000 in just the two-and-a-half years since my transplant. We will beat this disease and make lung transplants the last resort, not the *only* resort.

September is now Pulmonary Fibrosis Awareness Month. The proclamation has been made in BC and will be made in Ontario in September 2012. Soon it will be Canada-wide. This will give greater awareness to this dreadful disease and help make a cure possible. Without us establishing the Canadian Pulmonary Fibrosis Foundation, this would not have been possible.

I have made so many new friends since my transplant, both from my visits to rehab and numerous medical appointments at Toronto General, and through the Canadian Pulmonary Fibrosis Foundation, helping those who have been diagnosed, those who so often do not know where to go for answers. I have found people who want to volunteer, even if they are sick themselves, and have become friends with them. This journey has brought me new life in so many ways.

I was asked once if, now that I had new lungs, I would give up on the Foundation. I intend to go on fighting this disease and providing support for as long as I can, without risking the great gift I have been given. I truly feel I have no choice, and luckily Heather agrees.

Thank you to all those doctors and researchers who worked to help me and continue to help others who get this awful disease. As the population ages, the number of people being diagnosed with IPF is rising, and the disease is becoming better known to the medical profession as a whole. Improved techniques will ensure early diagnosis and allow the time needed for better outcomes. The work of the Foundation in increasing awareness translates into more people wanting to help us in our efforts.

I particularly thank those generous people who donate their organs to help others. Eight lives are saved from every donor and 75 other lives are positively affected.

I would like to extend a very special thank you to my donor who so selflessly signed the organ donor card, and to the loving family who honoured those wishes and gave me life.

About the Author

Robert Davidson was born in London, England in May 1947 and moved to Canada with his wife Heather in 1973.

Robert is a Chartered Accountant and Trust and Estate Practitioner and a fellow of The Institute of Chartered Accountants in England & Wales. He worked with various CA firms in London before joining Price Waterhouse in Toronto. After a 9 year spell as the CFO of a large private company he opened his own tax practice in Markham Ontario, running that until January 2010 when Idiopathic Pulmonary Fibrosis made it impossible to service his clients.

Robert founded the Canadian Pulmonary Fibrosis Foundation in late October 2009, just 3 months before his life-saving double lung transplant on January 30, 2010.

Robert and his wife live in Markham Ontario. He has two sons. Mark, who also lives in Markham with his wife, Alyshia and new baby daughter Alexis. His other son, Matthew, lives in Neurenberg, Germany where he works with Adidas and is marrying Gemma there in June 2013.

CPSIA information can be obtained
at www.ICGtesting.com
Printed in the USA
BVHW072034251218
536377BV00001B/90/P